# *Review of Microbiology*

**Vaneet Arora**
MD (Microbiology)

**Ranjana Arora**
MD (Microbiology)



PEEPEE
PUBLISHERS AND DISTRIBUTORS (P) LTD.

**Review of Microbiology**

*Published by*
**Pawaninder P. Vij**

Peepee Publishers and Distributors (P) Ltd.
*Head Office:* 160, Shakti Vihar, Pitam Pura
Delhi - 110 034 (India)

**Correspondence Address:**

**7/31, First Floor**
**Ansari Road, Daryaganj, Post Box-7243**
**New Delhi-110 002 (India)**

Ph: 65195868, 23246245, 9811156083

*e-mail:* peepee160@yahoo.co.in

*e-mail:* peepee160@rediffmail.com

*e-mail:* peepee160@gmail.com

**www.peepeepub.com**



*First Edition:* 2005
*Reprint:* **2009**

**ISBN:** 81-88867-055-1

*Printed at*
Lordson, C-5/19, Rana Pratap Bagh, Delhi-110007

*To*

*Mr. D.D. Arora*

*who has been and will always be*

*with us to show the right way to do*

*the right things*

# Preface

This book is mainly intended for undergraduate and postgraduate students of microbiology and anyone interested in infectious diseases, especially anyone appearing in the post-graduate medical admission tests of All India, different states, PGI Chandigarh, AIIMS, JIPMER, DNB, UPSC and MCI screening test for Foreign graduates etc.

Microbiology is one subject, which is considered boring by most and tough to remember by many, whereas the fact is, if presented well this can be one of the most interesting subjects. Knowledge and understanding of Microbiology not only helps in answering direct questions but also forms the basis of infectious diseases. This significantly adds on to the number of correct answers in clinical subjects especially medicine, pediatrics, ophthalmology, otorhinolaryngology etc. With the change in pattern of questions to clinical pattern especially in AIPG and AIIMS knowledge of clinical microbiology has become critical in reaching the diagnosis and more importantly correct answer to the question. This book aims to provide you with high yielding information in an uncomplicated fashion to help improve your performance.

This book is structured into eight sections. First six focus on different disciplines of microbiology namely, general microbiology, bacteriology, virology, mycology, parasitology and immunology. These are followed by a section summarizing the high frequency points or "the pearls" that you can read through and revise in a few minutes and be assured to answer majority of microbiology multiple choice questions. There is a section on MCQs at the end of the book followed by explanations. These will help you understand the reasoning for the answers to the MCQs without wasting time surfing various topics or books.

Based on our experience, some guidelines help in optimizing time without compromising on results:

- All parts of microbiology carry the same weightage in entrance exams. Therefore focus on those parts first which will require less time while give you a better yield. These are virology, mycology and immunology.
- Classification forms the basis of microbiology. Remember the common features of the group and names of members that belong to the group. All members of any taxonomic group will have same features. So you will not have to remember all features for all organisms independently. Focus on classification, general, as well as for bacteria, fungi, viruses, parasites.
- Focus on topics of current importance, those "in news" like SARS, Avian flu, or fashionable topics like HIV/AIDS, emerging diseases or opportunistic infections.
- Never leave the last few chapters of a book. For example, in bacteriology, it would be advisable to start from the back. Topics like Rickettsia, Mycoplasma, Chlamydia, Spirochetes will surely appear in questions while you may have been exhausted by the time you are through with Staphylococcus, Streptococcus, Corynebacteria..............., so on so forth.

Although, we have made our best efforts to ensure that the information provided in this book is accurate and updated, in this ever evolving field, no one can boast of being infallible. Therefore, we encourage all readers and critics to kindly inform us about any deficiencies. Any suggestions to improve the book will be most welcome.

**Vaneet Arora**
**Ranjana Arora**
email: ranjanavaneet@yahoo.com

# Contents

1. General Microbiology ........................... 1
2. Bacteriology ........................................ 37
3. Immunology ........................................ 178
4. Medical Mycology ............................... 197
5. Parasitology ........................................ 211
6. Virology ............................................... 234
7. High Frequency Points ........................ 273
8. Practice Questions ................................ 289
*Answers and Explanations* .................. *307*

CHAPTER ONE

# General Microbiology

**Microbiology** is the study of living organisms ('micro-organisms' or 'microbes'), simple in structure and small in size that includes bacteria, algae, fungi, protozoa and viruses.

> **'Pure'** microbiology concerns the organisms themselves.
> **'Applied'** microbiology concerns the effect of the micro-organisms on other living beings, when they act as pathogens or commensals, or on their inanimate environment, when they bring about chemical changes in it.

## HISTORICAL FACTS

- **Antonie van Leeuwenhoek** (1632-1723): Dutch lens-maker who was first to see and described micro-organisms
- **Louis Pasteur** (1822-1895) **Father of Micro-biology**
  - Established that fermentation was a result of microbial activity.
  - Described pasteurization techniques for disinfection of milk
  - Introduced techniques of sterilization. (hot air oven and autoclave).
  - Described varying growth needs of bacteria.
  - Coined the term vaccine, (attenuated cultures of Anthrax bacillus and proved that inoculation of such cultures in animals induced specific protection against anthrax)
  - Developed rabies vaccine.

- **Joseph Lister** (1827-1912) started the antiseptic regimen, to prevent surgical sepsis (1867).
- **Robert Koch** (1843-1910): **Father of Bacteriology.**
  - Established the fixing and staining of bacteria with aniline dyes.
  - Use of solid media to obtain pure cultures of bacteria.
  - Described *Vibrio cholerae*.
  - Discovered anthrax bacilli and anthrax vaccine.
  - Gave the aetiological role of tubercle bacilli.
  - Established Koch's postulates.

**Koch's postulates** are a set of conditions, which must be fulfilled to establish a relationship between the disease and isolate. These are:

1. The organism is regularly found in the lesion of the disease
2. It can be grown in pure culture outside the body of the host, for several generations
3. Such a culture will reproduce the disease in question when administered to a susceptible animal
4. It can be isolated from the lesions in the infected animal

- **Paul Ehrlich** (1878):
  - Demonstrated the acid-fastness of tubercle bacilli.
  - Also demonstrated the 'side chain theory' of antibody production.
- **Metchnikoff** (1883-91): Studied the cellular defence mechanisms.
- **Edward Jenner:** Use of Cowpox virus preparation for protection against smallpox.
- **Hansen**: Leprosy bacillus (1874).
- **Neisser**: Gonococcus (1879).
- **Ogston:** Staphylococcus (1881).
- **Loeffler:** Diphtheria bacillus (1884).
- **Walter Reed** (1902) proved first viral etiology (yellow fever).

- **Schaudinn** and **Hoffmann:** *Treponema pallidum* (1905).
- **Fleming:** Penicillin (1929).
- **Ruska:** Electron microscope (1934).
- **Jerne**: Natural selection theory of antibody synthesis (1955).
- **Burnet**: Clonal selection theory of antibody synthesis (1957).
- **Barbara McClintok**: Noble prize for discovery of transposons.

## CLASSIFICATION

Living beings are classified into 7 kingdoms:

- Animalia
- Plantae
- Fungi
- Protozoa
- Chromista

} Eukaryotes

- Archae
- Monera

} Prokaryotes

Viruses are not included in this classification as they are non-living

Major characteristics of eukaryotes and prokaryotes

| | *Eukaryotes* | *Prokaryotes* |
|---|---|---|
| Major groups | Algae, fungi, protozoa, plants and animals | Bacteria |
| Size (approx | >5µm | 1 × 3µm |
| Nuclear structure | Nuclear membrane | None |
| Chromosome type | Strands of DNA | Single, closed circular/ linear DNA. |
| Cytoplasmic structures | | |
| Mitochondria | + | – |
| Golgi apparatus | + | – |
| Endoplasmic reticulum | + | – |
| Ribosomes | 80S | 70S |
| Cytoplasmic membrane | +; sterols | +; No sterols |

*Contd.*

*Contd.*

| | | |
|---|---|---|
| Cell wall cellulose/chitin | -; or + with peptidoglycan (fungi) | Complex |
| Reproduction | Sexual/asexual | Binary fission. |
| Movement | Flagella complex when present | Flagella simple when present |

## MORPHOLOGY OF BACTERIA

Morphology and structure of the prokaryotic cell.

### Cell Wall

Prokaryotes (**except *Mycoplasma***) are surrounded by the cell wall, external to cytoplasmic membrane.

**Peptidoglycan** (unique to bacterial cell wall) provides tensile strength to maintain the structural integrity of the bacteria. It is a heteropolymer macromolecule consisting of alternating residues of N-acetylglucosamine (GlcNAc) and N-acetylmuramic acid (MurNAc) linked by b-1,4-glycosidic bonds. Short interpeptide bridges interlink these glycan chains to one another.

**Gram-positive cell wall**:

- 200-300 nm thick,
- Consists of **peptidoglycan and techoic acid** predominantly.

**Techoic acids** function as major surface antigens that help in serological categorisation of these bacteria. They also help in attachment of the bacterium to the mammalian cell, in strengthening the cell wall and transfer of magnesium ions through the cell wall.

**Gram-negative cell wall:**

- More complex.
- In addition to a **thinner peptidoglycan** layer, it also has an **outer membrane**.

The gram-negative cell wall is structurally quite different from the gram-positive cell wall. The peptidoglycan accounts for only 5-15% of the entire cell envelope. External to the peptidoglycan layer and attached to it by lipoproteins is the outer membrane.

**Outer membrane** has two leaflets:

- Inner one composed of **phospholipids**
- Outer leaflet is attached to another molecule unique to the bacterial wall, the **lipopolysaccharide.**

**Lipopolysaccharide** is **amphipathic** (one end of the molecule is hydrophilic and the other is hydrophobic) in character and consists of three components:

- Somatic antigen (O-specific, polysaccharide, hydrophilic).
- Core region (links 'O' with Lipid A)
- Lipid A (hydrophobic).

LPS is known as the **endotoxin.** Essentially all of the toxicity is based in the lipid A portion of LPS.

> Endotoxin (LPS) is produced only by gram-negative bacteria (as it is a part of the gram-negative cell wall and is released when cell wall is lysed)
> Exotoxins can be produced by all bacteria (gram-positive as well as gram-negative) as these are bacterial metabolites

In addition to LPS, the outer membrane also contains several important proteins that function in the selective transport of nutrients into the cell. These include:

- **Porins,** or **transmembrane proteins,** traverse the outer membrane and permit the transport of low MW hydrophilic molecules such as amino acids, sugars and ions. Some examples of porins are OmpC, OmpD, PhoE characteristic of *E. coli* and *S. typhimurium.*
- **Integral proteins** maintain its integrity.
- **Peripheral proteins** transport of molecules across the membrane.

| *Exotoxin* | *Endotoxin* |
|---|---|
| Proteins complexes | Proteins-polysaccharide-lipid |
| Heat labile stable | Heat stable |
| Secreted by cell; can be separated from cultures | Form part of gram-negative cell wall; obtained only by cell lysis |

*Contd.*

*Contd.*

| | |
|---|---|
| Action often enzymatic | No enzymatic action |
| Specific effect of each exotoxin | Fever, shock |
| Specific tissue affinity | No specific tissue affinity |
| Active in very minute doses (~ 1 mg) | Active only in large doses (~100 mg) |
| Highly antigenic | Weakly antigenic |
| Action specifically neutralized by antibody | Neutralization by antibody ineffective |
| Toxoids used as vaccines | Cannot be toxoided |
| Produced by both gram-positive and gram-negative bacteria | Cell wall of gram negative bacteria |

## Nucleoid

- The absence of a nuclear membrane in cells defines them as prokaryotes and different from the eukaryotic cells.
- The chromosome consists of a single, naked, closed circular DNA but when unfolded it spans a distance of 1 mm and occupies as much as 10% of the cell volume.
- Although majority of prokaryotes have **circular closed DNA**, some cells as *Borrelia burgdorferi* several streptomycetes have linear DNA.
- In addition to chromosome, some extrachromosomal genetic elements in the form of linear as well as circular plasmids have been found in some bacteria.
- The formation of a cell and its component parts requires the complex interaction between the cell's DNA and RNA. The end product of these interactions (DNA replication, transcription and translation), are the cell's proteins.

## Ribosomes and Polysomes

- Ribosomes are complex units comprised of ribonucleoproteins, which constitute 20% of the dry weight of a typical bacterium.
- These are the location of all bacterial protein synthesis. The functioning ribosomes translate (translation) the information encoded in mRNA into the amino acid sequences of proteins.

- During active growth and rapid protein synthesis, ribosomes are joined together as a **'beads on string'** known as **polysome**.
- Physical analysis reveals the ribosome to have a sedimentation rate of **70 Svedberg (S) units.**
- Chemical analysis reveals the ribosome to be composed of 50 different proteins associated with 3 types of RNA.
  - **Ribosomal (r) RNA** is composed of 3 subunits of sizes 23S, 16S and 5S. It is the most abundant of the RNAs, accounting for 80% of the total.
  - **Transfer (t) RNA** accounts for 15%
  - **Messenger (m) RNA** for only 4% of the total cellular RNA.

| The prokaryotic ribosomes (70S) differ from eukaryotic ribosomes, which are heavier (80S) |
|---|

### Intracellular Storage Material

Limitations in nutrients such as nitrogen, sulphur, phosphorus, acetate or existence of unfavourable growth conditions often result in the assimilation of excess available carbon into storage granules. These include:

### Polysaccharide

- Starch and glycogen are the most commonly recognized polysaccharide inclusions formed in bacteria.
  - *Clostridium* and *Neisseria* spp. store starch
  - *Bacillus, Escherichia, Micrococcus* and *Salmonella* store glycogen under growth stress conditions.

### Lipid

- The lipid storage granules are often polymers of β-hydroxy, short chain fatty acids to form poly-β-hydroxyalkanoic acid (PHA). Under conditions of oxygen or nitrogen limitation, PHA accumulates as granules that can be seen by selective stains only.

- *Bacillus, Clostridium, Pseudomonas and Rhodobacter* spp. are noted for PHA synthesis.

### Polyphosphate

- These inclusions are formed during generalized nutrient limitation, except phosphate. They are also referred to as **volutin** or **metachromatic** granules.
  - These are seen in *Corynebacterium* spp.

### Others

- Several species whose metabolism involves sulphur compounds accumulate **sulphur** as globules. Among these are the purple sulphur (*Chromatium)* phototrophic bacteria.
- Other complex intracytoplasmic inclusions are **magnetosomes** (composed of iron in various forms), **gas vesicles** (or vacuoles) in phototrophic organisms and **carboxysomes** (for carbon dioxide assimilation) in autotrophic organisms.

### Cytoplasmic Membrane

- The prokaryotic cytoplasmic (or cell) membrane encloses the cytoplasm.
- It is distinguished from the eukaryotic membrane by the **absence of sterols**, with the exception of *Mycoplasma*, which contains cholesterol in its membrane.
- **Selectively permeable** and is involved in the transport of molecules into and out of the cell.
- **Permeases** facilitate the passive diffusion or catalyse energy (in the form of ATP) dependent active transport.

There are at least three types of transport of solutes into a bacterial cell:

- **Primary active transport**, an active pump is used to assist in the movement of a specific solute across the cytoplasmic membrane against a concentration gradient.

- **Secondary active transport** involves specific carrier molecules for the transfer of selected solutes, primarily amino acids and proteins. In this co-transport, the specific carrier protein binds to the solute as well as to a proton or cation, and both are transported simultaneously.
- **Group translocation** involves the alteration of the solute prior to its transport. It routinely involves transport of sugars (i.e. glucose, mannose, galactose) and is mediated by phosphotransferase.

- On electron microscopy, the inner leaflet of cytoplasmic membrane forms complex convolutions known as **mesosomes,** which participate in cell division and are associated with the DNA molecule during cell division.
  - **Septal mesosomes:** at sites of cross-wall formation
  - **Lateral mesosomes:** random fashion.

### Extracellular Polymers: Capsules and Slimes

- **Capsules**, majority of which are polysaccharides, are polymers tightly associated with the cell wall.
- **Slime layers** are represented as large amounts of extracellular polymer that appear to entrap the bacterial cells within it. Slime layers are not directly attached to the cell wall.
- **S layers** are crystalline structured, composed of identical protein or glycoprotein subunits and are routinely found associated with those bacteria that live in stressful or harsh microenvironments, e.g *Aeromonas* and *Campylobacter*.
  - The function of these extracellular, accessory structures is to **protect the cell** from harsh environmental stresses, including change in pH and temperature.
  - Several capsules are also known to **protect the cell from phagocytic activity** by polymorph nuclear leucocytes.

- Capsules in several species assist them to adhere to both mammalian cells and other bacteria (i.e. **coaggregation**).
- The capsules of oral streptococci such as *Streptococcus mutans* and *Streptococcus salivarius* function to **attach** these bacteria to both hard (i.e. tooth resulting in caries) and soft tissue (i.e. mucosal surfaces).
- In some instances, bacterial capsules are associated with **increased virulence** as in case of *Streptococcus pneumoniae.*
- Although the **majority** of prokaryotic capsules and slimes are **polysaccharide, some** bacteria synthesize high molecular weight **peptides** as capsules; *Bacillus anthracis* and *Yersinia pestis* are 2 examples.
- *Bacillus subtilis* synthesizes a heteropolypeptide capsule composed of D- and L-glutamic acid.

## Flagella

- Bacterial flagella are appendages that help the bacteria to swim through liquids (**organs of locomotion**) and, for some bacteria to swarm over solid surfaces.
- The number and arrangement of these have been used in bacterial categorisation.
- The flagella can be sheathed (e.g. *Vibrio*) and unsheathed or naked.
- A motile cell may swim at the rate of 1-5 mm/min.
- Chemically, the bacterial flagellum is composed of multiple copies of subunits consisting of a single protein, termed **flagellin.**
- A prokaryotic flagellum consists of 3 major components:
  - Long semi-rigid, helical shaft or **filament** which rotates and propels the bacteria
  - Connecting **hook region**
  - **Basal body** embedded in the cytoplasmic membrane.

- Stabilization of the flagellum in the bacterial surface structures occurs by means of **flagellar rings** (one pair in gram-positive cells; 2 or more in gram-negative cells).
- Flagella are highly antigenic, and several of the immune response mounted by the host systems are directed against the **flagellar H antigens**.
- In spirochaetes, the flagella do not protrude to the external environment, but are rather located within the outermost layers of the cells; these are termed as the **endoflagella**.

| *Type of flagella* | *Flagellar arrangement* | *Example* |
|---|---|---|
| Atrichous | No flagella | *Shigella, Klebsiella spp etc* |
| Monotrichous | One flagellum, each end | *Vibrio* |
| Amphitrichous | One/several flagella, each end | *Listeria* |
| Lophotrichous | Two/several flagella, one/either end | *Aquaspirillum Helicobacter, Campylobacter* |
| Peritrichous | Flagella surrounding cell | Motile members of *Enterobacteriaceae* family |
| Endoflagellum | Flagella in a sheath, not free | Spirochetes |
| Lateral flagella | | *Vibrio parahaemolyticus.* |

## Fimbriae and Pili

- Though terms fimbriae and pili are used interchangeably, generally:
  - **Fimbriae** (fringes) describe the thin rod-like adhesins (in contrast to the thicker helical flagella) that emerge from the cell wall. Those fimbriae, which are involved in adherence to mammalian cell, are known as **type-specific fimbriae**. These play a role in the virulence of several pathogenic bacteria. They also provide the pathogens with specific adherence properties.

- **Pili** (hairs) routinely describe the very long, flexible, rod-like structures that also emerge from the cell wall and are involved in bacterial conjugation. The **sex pili** are involved in the formation of conjugation bridges between donor and recipient bacteria during conjugation.

- Fimbriae may be 3-25 nm in diameter and a single cell may be covered with as few fimbriae as 10 and as many as 1000.
- Pili and fimbriae are composed of a single protein subunit, **pilin**.
- Some specialized fimbriae help in motility, e.g. in *Eikenella.*

### Types of Motility

| *Descriptive term* | *Example* | *Cause of movement* |
|---|---|---|
| Darting | *Vibrio cholerae* | Polar flagella |
| Stately | Motile members of *Enterobacteriaceae* family (e.g. *E. coli, Salmonella, proteus*) | Peritrichous flagella |
| Writhing | Aerobic Spore Bearers (*Bacillus*) | Flagella |
| Twitching | *Eikenella* | Fimbriae |
| Gliding | *Capnocytophaga,* | Fimbriae |
| | *Cytophaga, Mycoplasma* | Unclear |
| Cork screw | Spirochetes | Endoflagella |
| Tumbling | *Listeria monocytogenes* | Amphitrichous Flagella |

Common bacterial exotoxins

| *Bacteria* | *Disease* | *Mode of action* |
|---|---|---|
| *Staphylococcus aureus* | 1. Toxic | Superantigen; binds to classII MHC and T cell receptor; induces Il-1 and IL-2 |
| | 2. Scalded skin syndrome | Protease that cleaves desmoglein in desmosomes |
| *Streptococcus pyogenes* | Scarlet fever | Superantigen; similar to staphylococcal toxic shock syndrome |

*Contd.*

*Contd.*

| | | |
|---|---|---|
| *Escherichia coli* | 1. Watery diarrhoea | Labile toxin stimulates adenylate cyclase by ADP-ribosylation; stable toxin stimulates guanylate cyclase |
| | 2. Bloody diarrhoea | Verotoxin in cytotoxic to enterocytes by degrading 28S ribosomal RNA |
| *Vibrio cholerae* | Cholera | Stimulates adenylate cyclase by ADP ribosylation |
| *Bordetella pertussis* | Whooping cough | Stimulates adenylate cyclase by ADP ribosylation; inhibits chemokine receptor |
| *Corynebacterium diphtheriae* | Diphtheria | Inactivates EF-2 by ADP ribosylation |
| *Clostridium tetani* | Tetanus | Blocks release of inhibitory neurotransmitter glycine by proteolytic cleavage of releasing proteins |
| *Clostridium perfringens* | Gas gangrene | Alpha toxin is a lecithinase |
| *Clostridium botulinum* | Botulism | Blocks release of acetylcholine by proteolytic cleavage of releasing proteins |
| *Clostridium difficile* | Pseudomembranous | Exotoxin B is cytotoxic to enterocytes by disaggregating actin filaments |
| *Bacillus anthracis* | Anthrax | Edema factor is an adenylate cyclase; lethal factor is a protease that cleaves MAP kinase, which is required for cell division |

## BACTERIAL GROWTH, ISOLATION AND IDENTIFICATION

### Bacterial Growth Requirements

In order for bacterial cells to grow, they must be provided with all of the chemical elements needed for the synthesis of the new cellular material. They require an appropriate temperature, gaseous atmosphere and nutritional provision. Bacteria are divided into 3 classes based on their oxygen requirements:

1. **Strict aerobes** grow only in the presence of oxygen (e.g. *Bacillus*).
2. **Strict anaerobes** grow only in the absence of oxygen. (e.g. *Clostridium*).
3. **Facultative organisms** (or **facultative anaerobes)** grow under aerobic and anaerobic conditions, though usually better in presence of oxygen. (e.g. *Enterobacteriaceae).*

**Microaerophilic** organisms grow best under a pressure of oxygen less than that of the atmosphere (2-3% $O_2$) (e.g. *Helicobacter*).

**Capnophilic** organisms grow best with 5-10% $CO_2$ for their growth (e.g. Pneumococci, meningococci, *H. influenzae*).

**Psychotropic** organisms grow at low temperatures, e.g. 2-5°C, and usually have a temperature optimum in the range 20-30°C.

**Mesophilic** organisms grow within the range 10-45°C and have a temperature optimum between 30 and 40°C.

**Thermophilic** organisms grow poorly or not at all at 37°C and have a temperature optimum between 50 and 60°C.

## Growth of Bacteria

### *Bacterial Nutrition and Culture of Bacteri*

- A **minimal medium** is one that contains the simplest chemical composition needed to support the growth of an organism. Bacteria have numerous nutritional needs that include different gases, water, various ions, nitrogen, and sources of carbon and energy. In the lab, nutrients are incorporated into culture media on or in which bacteria are grown. Since different pathogenic bacteria have different nutritional requirements, various types of culture media have been developed for use in diagnostic microbiology.

- Bacteria with complex nutritional needs requiring exceptional media components are said to be **fastidious** while those with basic nutritional needs are **non-fastidious.**

*Culture Media*

Growth media are used in either of two phases:

**Liquid broth:** Nutrients are dissolved in broth and growth is indicated by a change in the broth's turbidity. At least $10^6$ bacteria per millilitre of broth are needed for turbidity to be detected by the naked eye.

**Solid agar:** Are made by adding a solidifying agent to the nutrients and water.

- Agarose, the most common solidifying agent, has a unique property of melting at high temperatures (95° C) but resolidifying only after its temperature falls below 50° C.
- It is derived from certain sea weeds and is bacteriologically inert.
- It has no nutritive value and is used to solidify liquid media.

The media can be classified in many ways according to their phases, function or complexity. The various types of media are:

- **Basal media:** They include peptone water and nutrient broth, which are the most basic media used in the study of the common pathogenic bacteria. Nutrient broth includes peptone along with meat extracts. If 1-2% agar is added for solidification, it becomes nutrient agar.
- **Enriched media:** They are prepared to meet the nutritional requirement of fastidious organisms by addition of substances such as blood, serum and egg to a basal medium. Important examples include:
  - Blood agar for isolation of *Streptococcus*, *Staphylococcus*.

  - Chocolate agar for isolation of *Neisseria* and *Haemophilus*.
  - Bordet-Gengou for *Bordetella.*
  - Loeffler's serum slope for the isolation of *C. diphtheriae.* (There is a debate as to whether or not LSS is enriched, some people call it nutritionally deficient medium).
- **Enrichment media**: **Liquid media** that inhibit the growth of unwanted (commensals/ non-pathogenic) bacteria and supports the growth of wanted (pathogenic) bacteria from specimens from contaminated sites. Important examples are:
  - Tetrathionate and selenite broth for *Salmonella* and *Shigella*
  - Alkaline peptone water for *V. cholerae*.

  Also used for enhancing the growth of any bacteria in specimen from normally sterile sites like blood or CSF. Examples are:
  - Brain heart infusion broth
  - Glucose citrate broth
  - Bile broth.
- **Selective media**: **Solid media** that inhibit the growth of unwanted bacteria but permits the growth of required bacteria in the form of colonies. Important examples of this type of media are:
  - Desoxycholate citrate agar (DCA) for *Salmonella* and *Shigella*,
  - Wilson and Blair medium for *Salmonella*
  - Potassium tellurite blood agar for *Corynebacterium diphtheriae*
  - TCBS for *Vibrio.*
- **Indicator media or differential media**: When a substance added to a medium produces a visible change in the medium following the growth of a particular organism, it is called an indicator or differential medium. For example,
  - **MacConkey medium** contains lactose and an indicator, neutral red which turns red in acidic conditions. Those bacteria, which utilize lactose,

produce acid, which turns neutral red to change colour to red. Hence, lactose-fermenters (e.g. *E.coli, Klebsiella*, etc.) produce pink colonies on this medium as compared to non-lactose-fermenters (e.g. *Salmonella, Shigella, Proteus, Vibrio, Pseudomonas*, etc.), which produce colourless colonies.

- **Transport media:** Used to preserve the viability of the pathogen during the transport of the clinical sample from the hospital to the laboratory. Important examples are:
  - **Cary Blair medium** (known as **universal transport medium**)
  - Buffered glycerol saline
  - Amie's transport medium
  - Stuart's transport media for respiratory specimens.
  - Venkatraman- Ramakrishnan **(VR) fluid** for vibrios

The commonly used media available for routine diagnostic bacteriology are summarised below:

| *Medium* | *Primary purpose* |
|---|---|
| Bile esculin agar (BEA) | Differential isolation of *Enterococci* |
| Blood agar | Cultivation of fastidious organisms (enriched medium), determination of haemolytic reactions. |
| Bordet-Gengou agar | Isolation of *Bordetella pertussis.* |
| Buffered charcoal-yeast extract agar (BCYE) | Enrichment for *Legionella* spp. |
| Cefoperazone, vancomycin, amphotericin (CVA) medium | Selective for isolation of Campylobacter spp. |
| Cefsulodin-irgasan-novobiocin (CIN) agar | Selective for isolation of *Yersinia* spp. |
| Chocolate agar | *Haemophilus* spp and pathogenic *Neisseria* spp. |
| Columbia colistin-nalidixic acid (CNA) agar | Selective isolation of gram-positive cocci. |
| Cystine-tellurite blood agar | Isolation of *C. diphtheriae.* |
| MacConkey agar | Isolation and differentiation of lactose fermenting and non-lactose-fermenting enteric bacilli. |

*Contd.*

*Contd.*

| | |
|---|---|
| MacConkey sorbitol agar | For selection and differentiation of *E. coli* O157:H7 in stool specimen. |
| Mannitol salt agar | Selective isolation of *Staphylococcus*. |
| New York City (NYC) agar | Selective for *Neisseria gonorrhoeae* |
| Potassium Tellurite Blood agar | Selective for *C. diphtheriae* |
| Salmonella-Shigella (SS) agar | Selective for *Salmonella* and *Shigella* spp. |
| Skirrow agar | Selective for *Campylobacter* spp. |
| Thayer-Martin agar | Selective for *N. gonorrhoeae* and *N.meningitidis* |
| Thiosulphate citrate-bile salts (TCBS) agar | Selective and differential for vibrios. |
| Wilson Blair medium | Selective for *Salmonella* (used for stool samples) |
| Xylose lysine desoxy-cholate (XLD) agar | Isolation and differentiation of *Salmonella* and *Shigella* from other gram-negative enteric bacteria. |

## Bacterial Metabolism

### *Bacterial Growth Curve*

Bacteria multiply by **binary fission**. The time for a division cycle to be completed is known as the **generation time.**

- Generation time of *E. coli* is ~20 minutes
- Generation time of *M. tuberculosis* is ~20 hours
- Generation time of *M. leprae* is ~20 days

The rate of increase in bacterial number (or mass) is exponential (**logarithmic**) since the population doubles with each generation. If the bacteria are growing at a constant rate, then a plot of the cell number or mass against time results in an **exponential curve**.

The growth phases and the growth curve

- **The lag phase**: When an inoculum of cells is transferred to a growth medium, a delay may take place before measurable growth occurs. This lag phase is a period when the bacterial cells are adjusting to the new growth conditions. During this phase, the cells increase in size before cell division can take place. **Morphological, biochemical and antimicrobial susceptibility patterns** are best observed towards the end of lag phase.

- **The exponential (logarithmic) growth phase:** Once the cells have adjusted to the new growth conditions, the culture enters the exponential or logarithmic growth phase where cells have approximately the same generation time. During this phase, the cells exist in different stages of division cycle. This stage lasts till the nutrients become limiting or the accumulation of some produce becomes toxic. **Exotoxin production** is the maximum in the log phase.
- **The stationary phase**: Eventually the stationary phase is reached, a period when measurable growth ceases. During this phase, the increase in the number of cells is balanced by the decrease in their number. This occurs due to the continued depletion of nutrients, change in pH and depletion of the energy source. **Endotoxin levels** are the highest in the stationary phase.
- **The death phase**: Some bacteria retain viability upon reaching the stationary phase while others rapidly lose viability and enter a death phase. A variety of reasons cause this loss of viability. There is a complete depletion of reserve foods that lead to cell starvation, some bacteria produce autolysins that cause their own lysis.

### Continuous Cultures of Bacterial Cells

Chemostat is a device, which is used to maintain the growth of bacteria in a constant exponential growth rate. This is done by continuously replacing the used medium with new sterile medium and maintaining constant growth conditions.

## BACTERIAL GENETICS

Genetics is the **study of genes**, their structures, organizations and expression. The characteristics expressed by a cell are referred to as its **phenotype**. The set of genes found in any particular cell constitutes its **genome**, which consists of a large circular DNA molecule, the bacterial chromosome and possibly one or more smaller circular DNA molecules called **plasmids**.

### Mutation

Mutation is a permanent change in the base sequence of DNA, which may or may not be expressed phenotypically. Mutations can be:

- **Spontaneous:** Occur in the absence of a specific treatment to generate them .
- **Induced:** Deliberately to provoke changes in the base sequence of the DNA. This can be achieved by:
  - Chemical treatment with known mutagens
  - Irradiation with ultraviolet or $\gamma$-rays.

With the use of recombinant DNA technology, it has become possible to target mutations into particular nucleotide sequences, a procedure termed as **site-specific mutagenesis**.

Mutations can be divided into 2 groups:

- **Microlesions (Point mutations):** Point mutations are of two classes:
- **Base pair substitutions:** Those mutants in which a single base pair has been altered and can be subdivided into:
  - **Transition,** which is more common, occurs when one purine is replaced by another purine and a pyrimidine is replaced by a different pyrimidine. Nitrous acid and powerful alkylating agents as ethylmethane sulphonate (EMS) can induce transition.

- **Transversion** is that base pair mutation in which a purine is replaced be a pyrimidine or vice-versa.

Point mutations are in general **revertible,** i.e. a second mutational event at the same site can precisely reverse the first mutation and restore the original base sequence.

- **Frame-shift mutations:** They are those in which one or a few base pairs have been added to or removed from the DNA Acridine dyes (e.g. proflavine) induce frame-shift mutation.
  - **Ames test** is a well-known test, used to test chemicals to determine if they are mutagenic (and so, potentially carcinogenic).
  - A **missense mutation** gives rise to a codon that specifies an amino acid different from the originally encoded. This could result in a **conditional-lethal mutation,** i.e. the mutation is lethal but only at higher temperatures.
  - Point mutation may change a codon from one specifying an amino acid to **nonsense codons,** one specifying termination of protein synthesis, namely UAG, UAA or UGA, because they do not code for an amino acid. The introduction of a nonsense codon into an early gene of an operon is called **polar mutation.**

- **Macrolesions**

  Alteration of DNA involving large numbers of base pairs is of 4 types:
- **Deletions**
  - **Duplications**
  - **Inversions**
  - **Additions**

- UV-induced mutations
  - Mutations may be induced by ultraviolet (UV) light and the most frequent mutation induced in the DNA by UV irradiation is the formation of **pyrimidine dimers** (most commonly thymidine dimers).

– If UV treated cells are immediately exposed to visible light of wavelength 300-400 nm, both mutation frequency and lethality are greatly reduced, a phenomenon called **photoreactivation**. The visible light treatment activates an enzyme, **photolyase** that hydrolyses the cyclobutane ring, reversing the reaction.

### Mobile Genetic Elements: Insertion Sequences and Transposons

- **Insertion sequences** (or IS elements) and **transposons** are now known to be one type of class of genetic elements that can insert into different sites on the same or on different DNA molecules.
- They are common in bacterial plasmids and are normal components of many, if not all, bacterial chromosomes.
- Because of their ability to insert into a large number of sites, both on the bacterial chromosomes and on the plasmid, they assumed the popular name of **'jumping genes'.**
- Because of their ability to insert into replicons almost randomly, transposons have been exploited as mutagens.

### Integrons and gene cassettes

- In addition to plasmids and transposable elements, bacteria have another system for gene dissemination, namely, **integrons.**
- Integrons are site-specific recombination systems that mediate the movement of small DNA elements called **gene cassettes (or pathogenicity islands).**
- They have a role to play in transferring resistance genes for antibiotics as aminoglycosides, β-lactams, tetracycline as well as virulence factors/ genes encoding toxins, e.g. cholera toxin and accessory toxin genes.

## Acquisition of New Genes in Bacteria

Four mechanisms of gene transfer have been described for bacteria, although not all apply to a particular bacterial species or strain; these are **transformation, transduction, conjugation** and **cell-cell fusion.**

### Transformation

- **Acquisition of DNA** by a bacterium from its environment and incorporation in its genome is known as transformation.
- **Griffith first** demonstrated transformation in 1928.

> **Griffith experiment**: *Streptococcus pneumoniae* in capsulated form is extremely virulent for mice, whereas the non-capsulated variants are avirulent. The virulence of the organism is due to polysaccharide capsule. Mutant strains that have lost their ability to synthesize capsule arise spontaneously and show rough (R) colonies on blood agar as compared to smooth (S) colonies of capsulated strains. Griffith mixed live noncapsulated cells that had produced a capsule of one antigenic type with heat-killed smooth cells of a different capsular type. Neither preparation alone had caused disease in the mice, but the mixture of the two preparations was lethal. He was able to isolate live capsulated pneumococci from the blood of the mice. It was shown later in 1944, by **Avery, MacLeod and McCarty**, that the transforming principle was DNA, which was released from the heat, killed bacteria and was able to supply the genetic information needed to produce the new type of capsule

### Transduction

- Transfer of a portion of DNA from one bacterium to another **by bacteriophages** is known as transduction.
- Two forms have been described:
  - **Generalized transduction** involves any part of the donor genome
  - **Restricted transduction,** specific sequences are transduced.

## Conjugation

- Conjugation is the term used to describe the transfer of DNA **directly from one bacterial cell to another** by a mechanism that requires cell-to-cell contact.
- It is a **major mechanism of transfer of drug resistance** and is more common amongst gram-negative bacteria.
- Bacterial conjugation was first described in 1946 by **Lederberg and Tatum** when testing pairs of mutant strains of *E coli* K12 for DNA transfer and recombination.
- Recombination due to bacterial conjugation is not the result of sexual reproduction with equal participation of both the parents in the zygote formation. Rather, only a small amount of DNA from the 'male' (**donor**) parent is incorporated into the offspring (**recombinants**) which otherwise showed all the characteristics of the 'female' (**recipient**) parent.
- The capacity to donate genetic information (DNA) depends upon the possession of the **F (fertility) factor.** Strains, which lose this F-factor, become infertile, but they can gain fertility by contact with an F-carrying ($F^+$) strain. The F-factor is now known as the **conjugative plasmid.**
- The donor and the recipient cells must contact each other for conjugation to occur and this contact is directed by thin protein filaments on the donor cell called **conjugative** or **'sex' pili.**
- The fertility or F-factor contains the genetic information necessary for the synthesis of sex pilus and for self-transfer, but it does not possess any other genetic markers as drug resistance.

## High Frequency of Recombination (HFR) and F Formation

- F-factor has the ability to integrate in the host chromosome.

- Such cells with the F-factor stably integrated into the chromosome are called **HFR** strains, because when these act as donors, chromosomal genes are carried into all recipients and high numbers of recombinants can be recovered.
- F-factor can revert from the bound state to free state, and during this process can carry with it some chromosomal genes. Such F-factor possessing chromosomal genes is known as **F′ (F prime) factor**.
- When this F′ mates with a recipient cell, it also transfers the host genes incorporated in the F-factor along with the F-factor DNA. This process resembles transduction and is known as **sex-duction**.

### Plasmids

- Plasmids are extrachromosomal, autonomous DNA molecules found in many bacterial cells.
- The word 'autonomous' here means self-governing, in that the plasmids use the replication enzymes of the host to ensure their own propagation, but retain control over replication.
- The term **episome**, which was a synonym for plasmids in the past, are defined as genetic elements that could exist and be replicated in either of 2 modes, autonomously or as part of a co-integrate with the bacterial chromosome.
- Though the plasmids represent only a fraction of the prokaryotic genetic pool, the genes they carry determine many features expressed by the bacteria, which include resistance to antibiotics and many heavy metals, virulence and metabolic activities.

### Resistance Plasmid or R-factor

It consists of two parts:

- **Resistance transfer factor (RTF):** responsible for conjugal transfer.
- **Resistance determinants (r)**: code for resistance against various drugs.

- As many as eight or more r determinants can be carried on each plasmid, and thus, resistance to eight or more drugs can be transferred simultaneously.
- Sometimes RTF dissociates from r determinants. Those plasmids that lack RTF and possess only r determinants are known as **non-conjugative or nonself-transmissible plasmids**.
- Those plasmids, which possess both RTF and r determinants are known as **conjugative or self-transmissible plasmids**.
- Plasmid mediated drug resistance is seen in various pathogenic organisms as *E. coli, K. pneumoniae, Proteus, Salmonella, Shigella, Pseudomonas* and *Vibrio*.
- Transferable drug resistance involves all antibiotics in common use.
- Plasmid mediated drug resistance can spread in the community due to indiscriminate use of antibiotics.

Mechanism of action of common antibacterial and antifungal agents

| *Mechanism of action* | *Drugs* |
|---|---|
| Inhibition of cell wall synthesis | |
| • Inhibition of cross-linking (transpeptidation) of peptidoglycan | Penicillins, cephalosporins, imipenam, aztreonam, vancomycin |
| • Inhibition of other steps in peptidoglycan synthesis | Cycloserine, bacitracin |
| • Inhibition of β-glucan synthesis | Caspofungin |
| Inhibition of protein synthesis | |
| • Action on 50S ribosomal subunit | Chloramphenicol, erythromycin, clindamycin, linezolid |
| • Action on 30S ribosomal subunit | Tetracyclines, aminoglycosides |
| Inhibition of nucleic acid synthesis | |
| • Inhibition of nucleotide synthesis | Sulfonamides, trimethoprim |
| • Inhibition of DNA synthesis | Quinolones |
| • Inhibition of mRNA synthesis | Rifampicin |

*Contd.*

*Contd.*

| | |
|---|---|
| Alteration of cell membrane function | |
| • Antibacterial activity | Polymyxin |
| • Antifungal activity | Amphotericin B, nystatin, ketoconazole |
| Other mechanisms | |
| • Inhibits mycolic acid synthesis | Isoniazid |
| • Act as electron sink (effective against anaerobes) | Metronidazole |
| • Inhibits synthesis of arabinogalactan | Ethambutol |
| • Inhibits fatty acid synthetase | Pyrazinamide |
| • Prevents formation of mitotic spindles by binding to tubulin | Griseofulvin |

Mechanisms of drug resistance

| *Mechanism* | *Important example* | *Drugs commonly affected* |
|---|---|---|
| Inactivate drug | Cleavage by β-lactamase | Penicillins, Cephalosporins |
| Modify drug target in bacteria | Mutation in Penicillin Binding Proteins (PBPs) | Penicillins |
| | Mutation in protein in 30S ribosomal subunit | Aminoglycosides,e.g. streptomycin |
| | Replace alanine with lactate in peptidoglycan | Vancomycin |
| | Mutation in DNA gyrase | Quinolones |
| | Mutation in RNA polymerase | Rifampicin |
| | Mutation in catalase peroxidase | Isoniazid |
| Reduce permeability of drug | Mutation in porin proteins | Penicillins, aminoglycosides |
| Export of drug from bacteria | Multidrug resistant pump (efflux pump) | Tetracyclines, sulfonamides, quinolones |

## General Approach to Diagnosis of an Infection

1. **Choose** the appropriate specimen on the basis of clinical presentation of the patient.

2. **Obtain** a specimen from the infected site. If the specimen is obtained away from the laboratory, it has to be transported safely and if required in an appropriate transport medium.
3. In the laboratory:
   a. **Gross examination**:
   Most important, as this may give important leads to the type of pathogen, e.g. CSF showing **cobweb** formation is possibly from tubercular meningitis; **bluish green pus** indicates *Pseudomonas aeruginosa*; stool may show **adult worms** or segments of worms depicting helminthic infestation, or presence of blood and/or mucus in stool would mean the processing should be done for dysentery causing organisms
   b. **Microscopy:**
   i. **Light microscopy** is the commonest microscopy done
      1. **Wet preparations**: For example **India ink** preparation of CSF which is a negative stain for capsulated organisms in CSF; **saline preparation** of stool for trophozoites of protozoa and ova/eggs of helminths; **iodine preparation** of stool for cysts of trophozoites
      2. **Fixed stained smears**: For examples
         a. **Gram stain**: Shape, size, arrangement; **differential stain** as this helps to differentiate bacteria into two groups Gram-negative or gram-positive
         b. **Acid-fast staining**: Ziehl-Neelson (ZN) staining for acid-fast organisms like *Mycobacteria, Nocardia* (*M. tuberculosis* is strongly acid-fast, can resist decolorization by 20% $H_2SO_4$; *M. leprae* upto 5% $H_2SO_4$; *Nocardia* upto 1%); Modified ZN staining or cold acid-fast staining known as **Kinyoun's** staining is done for oocysts of

*Cryptosporidium parvum* in stool of immunocompromised individuals with diarrhea

c. **Albert's staining**: **Metachromatic** staining done for *Corynebacterium diphtheriae*, shows metachromatic granules

ii. **Darkfield microscopy**: done for thin organisms like **spirochetes** which appear as bright objects against a dark background

iii. **Phase contrast microscopy**: also done for thin organisms and structures; uses special condenser to create a phase difference in the rays of light falling on the object

iv. **Electron microscopy**:
   1. **Transmission EM**: gives two-dimensional image; shows ultrastructure
   2. **Scanning EM**: shows three-dimensional image; surface topography

v. **Confocal microscopy**: uses special condensers used for reading microarrays

c. **Culture**: done on appropriate media at appropriate environment i.e. in the presence or absence of oxygen as required, and streaked on the media in such a manner as to obtain isolated colonies, i.e., a **'pure culture'.**

d. **Identify:** done by looking at colony morphology, appropriate biochemical tests and/or serotyping

e. **Antibiotic Susceptibility**

i. **Dilution methods**: Broth dilution or agar dilution. The results reported as "**Minimum inhibitory concentration**", which is defined as the lowest concentration of the drug that inhibits the growth of an organism. This helps in choice of both the drug and the dose required. MIC does not indicate whether the inhibited organisms are killed or have just stopped growing. For certain infections like endocarditis, the '**Minimum Bactericidal**

**Concentration'** has to be calculated. This is the lowest concentration of drug that kills the bacteria.

ii. **Disc diffusion methods**: Discs impregnated with different antibiotics are placed on the surface of agar plate and after incubation, diameter of zone of inhibition is measured. In **Kirby Bauer** method, the size of zone of inhibition is compared with standardized charts for different organisms and antibiotics. In **Stoke's** method, a control strain is plated along with the test strain for comparison on the same agar plate.

f. **Immunologic (serologic) testing**:
Antigen antibody reactions may be carried out to provide indirect evidence of an infection in the form of body's immune response **(antibody detection)** or **detection of antigens** of the organism. Presence of significant titers of **specific IgM antibody** is a good indicator of recent infection. Single titer of IgG is not useful in most situations. A **four-fold rise** in titre is a clear indication of infection, but this is usually a retrospective diagnosis as by 10-14 days when the rise in titer of antibodies is detected, patient may not have symptoms any more.
When corresponding antigen and antibody are allowed to interact, they combine, but this combination may not be visible to the naked eye. To make the antigen-antibody reaction visible, different carrier particles or indicator systems can be used, which provide the names to different serological reactions.

| *Serological test* | *Indicator system/carrier* |
|---|---|
| Latex agglutination | Latex particles |
| Haemagglutination | RBCs |
| Fluorescent immunoassay | Fluorescent dye |
| Radio immunoassay | Radioactive isotope |
| Enzyme immunoassay | Enzyme substrate reaction |

Common Serological tests

| *Test* | *Agent/Disease* | *Principle* |
|---|---|---|
| Widal test | Enteric fever | Tube agglutination |
| Blood grouping | | Slide agglutination |
| Serotyping of salmonellae | *Salmonella* | Slide agglutination |
| Lancefield grouping | Streptococci | Capillary precipitation |
| VDRL | Syphilis | Slide flocculation |
| Kahn's test | Syphilis | Tube flocculation |
| Wassermann reaction | Syphilis | Complement fixation test |
| Paul-Bunnell test | Infectious mononucleosis | Tube agglutination |
| ASLO | *Streptococcus pyogenes* | Neutralization |
| Cold agglutinin | *Mycoplasma* | Tube agglutination |
| Weil-Felix reaction | Rickettsial diseases | Tube agglutination |

Immunodiffusion (precipitation in gel)

| *Type* | *Name* | *Common use* |
|---|---|---|
| Single diffusion in one dimension | Oudin procedure | |
| Double diffusion in one dimension | Oakley-Fulthrope procedure | |
| Single diffusion in two dimensions | Radial immuno-diffusion | Measure amount of various Ig classes in patient serum; lab diagnosis of multiple myeloma |
| Double diffusion in two dimensions | Ouchterlony procedure | Comparison of different antigens for identical or cross-reacting components; Elek's test for diphtheria is a special variety |
| One-dimensional single electro-immunodiffusion | Rocket electro-phoresis | Quantitation of antigen |
| One-dimensional double electro-immunodiffusion | Counter immuno-electrophoresis | Detection of HBsAg. |

**g. Molecular methods**

These methods involve detection of nucleic acid can be done either by:

- **Non-amplification methods**: direct detection of nucleic acid in the specimen, e.g. DNA hybridization using DNA probes

- **Amplification methods**:
  - **Polymerase chain reaction (PCR)**: carried out in a thermocycler. The steps include:
    - **Denaturation** at 94°C: separation of strands
    - **Annealing** at 54°C: attachment of primer (specificity of the primer determines the accuracy of the PCR)
    - **Extension** at 72°C: polymerase becomes active and new strand is formed (Polymerase used is Taq polymerase derived from thermophilic organism *Thermus aquaticus.*

    The product is run in an agarose gel and watched for presence of amplified nucleic acid under UV light after staining with **ethidium bromide.**

  PCR is used in various forms:
  - **Nested PCR**: two sets of primers used sequentially to make diagnosis specific.
  - **Multiplex PCR**: Primers for multiple organisms put in the same PCR cycle, any one of those organisms present in the sample can be detected with just one PCR test, useful for CSF samples
  - **RT (Reverse transcriptase)-PCR**: Used for quantitation of viral copies, which is the best indicator for **prognosis and response to therapy** in HIV/AIDS and Hepatitis B or Hepatitis C.

- **Ligase chain reaction**: Amplification method but does not require thermocycler. Two pairs of primers which attach with the target nucleic acid adjacent to each other have to be selected. Has been used for *Chlamydia* and Mycobacteria.

Molecular methods (genotypic methods) are also used for **epidemiological typing/ strain differentiation.**

- **Randomly amplified polymorphic DNA (RAPD):** Also known as **Arbitrarily Primed (AP)-PCR**, an amplification method.
- **Pulsed field gel electrophoresis (PFGE):** Uses

restriction endonucleases; this is a non amplification method and also the gold standard for epidemiological typing.

## STERILIZATION AND DISINFECTION

**Sterilization**: Removal of all microorganisms (vegetative or spore) from an article, surface or medium

**Disinfection**: Destruction of all pathogenic organisms from an inanimate article/surface (some bacteria and spores survive).

**Antisepsis**: Removal of vegetative forms from animate surfaces/tissues like skin.

### Methods of Sterilization

*Heat-based methods:*

**Dry heat–Hot air oven**: 160°C for 1 hour. This method is used for glassware (e.g. Petri dishes, all-glass syringes), oils, wax, powders, and sharp surgical instruments.

**Moist heat–Autoclaving:** 121°C for 15 minutes at 15 pounds per square inch pressure. This method is the most widely used. Articles made of plastic, rubber, cotton can be sterilized by this method (e.g. gloves, masks, gowns, linen, cotton swabs, glass containers with rubber washer, catheters, test tube with cotton plugs, agar, blunt surgical instruments). Prions and coxiella survive at 121°C, these are killed at 134°C.

> Indicators of sterilization:
> Physical: thermocouples
> Chemical: Brownie's tapes
> Biological: Spores of *Bacillus stereothermophilus* (for autoclave) or spores of *Clostridium tetani* var niger (for hot air oven)

**Tyndallization:** 80°C for 30 minutes on three consecutive days with overnight incubation at 37°C in between. Method used for media containing egg or sera, e.g. LJ medium, Loeffler's serum slope.

- **Inspissation** is not a method of sterilization. It is a method of solidifying for media containing egg or serum. One time exposure at 80°C for 30 minutes
- **Pasteurization** is a method of disinfection of milk to get rid of pathogenic organism like *Mycobacterium bovis, Salmonella, Streptococcus, Listeria* and *Brucella*. It is not a method of sterilization. Can be done by
  - –Holder method: 63°C for 30 minutes followed by rapid cooling
  - –Flash method: 72°C for 15 seconds followed by rapid cooling.

### Filtration

For heat sensitive liquids like **sugar solutions, vaccines, serum, antibiotic solutions.**

Filters are of following types:

i. Candle filters—used for purification of water.
ii. Asbestos filters—have carcinogenic potential
iii. Sintered glass filters—brittle and expensive
iv. **Membrane filter–widely used for sterilization** and separation of particles on the basis of size.

### Radiation

Used for **mass or bulk sterilization** by manufacturers, e.g. disposable gloves, disposable needles, sutures and syringes.

**γ-rays** are used for sterilization known as **cold sterilization.**

UV rays act as surface disinfectants, used at entry of OT, nursery, ICU, restaurants.

### Chemical

Most chemicals act as disinfectants. Some can be used as chemical sterilants:

**Ethylene oxide**: Gaseous agent used for mass or bulk sterilization by manufacturers or big hospitals with large loads of material

**Glutaraldehyde**: Used for sterilization of endoscopes, bronchoscopes. Exposure time has to be overnight for sterilization. Exposure for 20-30 minutes provides high level disinfection.

### New Methods of Sterilization

**Low temperature steam formaldehyde (LTSF):** If the pressure of an environment is brought to below atmospheric level, the boiling point of formalin falls to 80°C. Steam at this temperature has better penetration than liquid form. This method is useful for heat sensitive articles.

**Gas plasma**: Utilizes oxygen radicals as means of sterilization. These radicals are formed by breaking down $H_2O_2$. Used for heat sensitive articles

**Microwaving**: Microwaves cause vibration and agitation of water molecules which strike each other to produce heat, which results in killing of organisms.

## DISINFECTANTS

1. **Alcohols**:
   Used mainly as skin antiseptics, no action on spores, 70 % alcohol works better than 100%. Isopropyl alcohol is preferred over ethyl alcohol .
   Methyl alcohol is effective against fungal spores and is used for treating cabinets and incubators. Methyl alcohol vapor is toxic and inflammable.
2. **Aldehydes**:
   **Formaldehyde**: Bactericidal, sporicidal and virucidal; used for preserving specimen. Formaldehyde gas is used for fumigating wards, OTs. It is irritant and toxic when inhaled.
   **Glutaraldehyde**: It is especially effective against tubercle bacilli, fungi and viruses. Less toxic and irritant than formaldehyde. Can be used for sterilization of corrugated rubber tubes, face-masks, endotracheal tubes, metal instruments and polythene tubing.
3. **Dyes** :
   a. aniline dyes
   b. acridine dyes.

Used as skin and wound antiseptics.
Aniline dyes are brilliant green, malachite green and crystal violet. Acridine dyes–Perflavine, Acriflavine

4. **Halogens:**
   - Iodine in aqueous and alcoholic solutions is used as skin antiseptic, especially useful prior to collection of samples for blood cultures.
   - Chlorine and hypochlorite–Markedly bactericidal, virucidal and effective against Hepatitis B and HIV. Chlorine used for water supplies, swimming pools.
   - Sodium hypochlorite (bleaching agent) is also known as the **universal disinfectant**
5. **Phenols**: Active against wide range of Gram + ve and Gram –ve bacteria and microbacteria. It has less activity against spores and viruses.
6. **Gases:**
   - **Ethylene oxide**
   - **Formaldehyde gas**
   - **Beta propiolactone** (BPL)

Tests done to check the effectiveness of disinfectants work on calculation of phenol coefficient, e.g. Rideal Walker test or Chick Martin test.

# CHAPTER TWO

# Bacteriology

## GRAM-POSITIVE BACTERIA

### GRAM-POSITIVE COCCI

### STAPHYLOCOCCI

#### Introduction

Staphylococci (derived from the Greek word *Staphyle*, meaning bunch of grapes) appear in clusters due to division in many planes. They are gram-positive cocci, catalase positive, non-motile, non-sporing and facultative anaerobes.

#### Classification

The family Micrococcaceae is composed of three genera: *Micrococcus, Planococcus* and *Staphylococcus*. Genus *Staphylococcus* contains nearly 32 species, and majority of infections caused in humans is by *Staphylococcus aureus.* Other common species are *S. epidermidis, S. saprophiticus, S.hominis, S. simulans* and *S. hemolyticus.*

#### Antigenic Structure

- **Peptidoglycan** and **Techoic acid** are the major components of the staphylococcal cell wall. The peptidoglycan amounts to about 50-60% of the dry weight and techoic acid is 30-50% of the dry weight.
  - Peptidoglycan plays an important role in maintaining the spherical shape of the cell.

- Techoic acid contributes to binding of antibodies, bacteriophages and lectins.

- **Protein A** is isolated from 90% of biotype strains isolated from man. It is a factor that plays a role in enhancement of virulence of the organism.
- **Capsular polysaccharide** is seen in some strains of *S. aureus (*though generally speaking staphylococci are noncapsulated). These strains are more virulent and relatively resistant to phagocytosis.
- **Slime** is a complex extracellular substance produced by many strains of *S. epidermidis.* Continued production of slime by a growing clone of cells attached to a polymer surface (e.g. an implanted catheter) results in encasement and formation of **biofilm** which may act as a penetration barrier for antibiotics.

## Pathogenicity

Pathogenicity or virulence determinants for *S. aureus*

### Cell-Wall Associated Factors

| |
|---|
| Capsule |
| Protein A |
| Peptidoglycan |
| Techoic acid |
| Clumping factor |

### Extracellular Factors

Staphylococcal extracellular proteins

| *Protein* | *Major biochemical and biological activities* |
|---|---|
| α-toxin (α-haemolysin) | Dermonecrotic, neurotoxic and cytotoxic. |
| β-toxin | Phospholipase C activity, especially for sphingomyelin and lysolecithin. |
| γ-toxin | Cytolytic for erythrocytes and leucocytes. |
| δ-toxin | Lyses erythrocytes. |
| Leucocidin | Cytolytic for leucocytes. |

*Contd.*

*Contd.*

| | |
|---|---|
| **Pyrogenic exotoxins (superantigens)** | |
| Enterotoxin A<br>Enterotoxin B<br>Enterotoxin C<br>Enterotoxin D<br>Enterotoxin E<br>Enterotoxin H | Gastrointestinal intoxication.<br>Mitogenic activity for T cells. |
| **Toxic Shock Syndrome Toxin 1(TSST-1)** | Toxic shock syndrome.<br>Mitogenic activity for T cells. |
| **Epidermolytic toxins** | |
| Exfoliatin A<br>Exfoliatin B | Staphylococcal scalded skin syndrome |
| **Fibrin forming and fibrinolytic enzymes** | |
| Staphylocoagulase (coagulase) | Clots plasma in the absence of $Ca^{2+}$.<br>Coagulase reacts with coagulase reacting factor (CRF) and the residual complex (staphylothrombin) converts fibrinogen to fibrin. |
| Staphylokinase | Binds to plasminogen and activates it to become the fibrinolytic enzyme plasmin. |
| **Bacteriolytic enzymes** | |
| Lysostaphin<br>Lipase<br>Nuclease<br>Urease<br>Hyaluronidase<br>Protease | |

## Clinical Disease

The clinical disease is primarily associated with *S. aureus*.

| | *Type of infections* | *Clinical presentation* |
|---|---|---|
| Superficial infections | Pyoderma (Impetigo) | Formation of vesicles of variable sizes. |
| | Folliculitis, furuncles (boils) and sties. | Infection of hair follicles. |
| | Abscesses and carbuncles. | Multiple, interconnected abscesses in hair follicles, sebaceous glands, surrounding tissues. |
| Deep infections | Osteomyelitis | Organism reaches bone via haematogenous route. |

*Contd.*

*Contd.*

| | | |
|---|---|---|
| | Pneumonia | Formation of lung abscess mostly in debilitated patients. |
| | Acute endocarditis | Usually in iv drug users or patients with prosthetic valves. ***S. epidermidis***—more common in **acute endocarditis.** ***Streptococcus viridans*** **group**—more common in **subacute endocarditis.** |
| | Arthritis, bacteremia, septicaemia, deep organ (brain, kidney, lung abscesses.) involvement. | Symptoms pertaining to systemic involvement. |
| **Staphylococcal toxin diseases** | Scalded skin syndrome (bullous impetigo) | Mainly in infants and children <5 years, exfoliation causes blisters that eventually rupture. |
| | Staphylococcal Scarlet fever | Nondesqamating erythematous rash. |
| **Staphylococcal food poisoning** | Staphylococcal enterotoxin | Vomiting and diarrhoea 1-5 hours after consumption of food contaminated with **staphylococcal enterotoxin** (and not the organisms). |
| Toxic Shock Syndrome | TSST-1 | Febrile illness that may progress to organ failure and death characterized by vomiting, diarrhoea, erythematous rash, muscle pain and hypotension. |

## Coagulase Negative Staphylococci

*S. epidermidis* causes
- Endocarditis in patients with prosthetic valves.
- Peritonitis in patients undergoing dialysis.
- Ventricular shunt infections.

*S. saprophiticus* causes
- Acute UTI in young women.

## Epidemiology

- *S. aureus* colonises the skin and mucous membranes of most of normal humans. The anterior nares is the most commonly populated site.
- It is also an important cause of nosocomial infection.
- Phage typing can be used to trace the source of staphylococcal infection.

## Laboratory Diagnosis

**Microscopy**: Clusters of gram-positive cocci in patients specimen is strongly suggestive of infections by staphylococci.

**Culture:** The specimen can be plated on blood agar for isolation of staphylococci. The media is inoculated and incubated at 37° C for 24 hours.

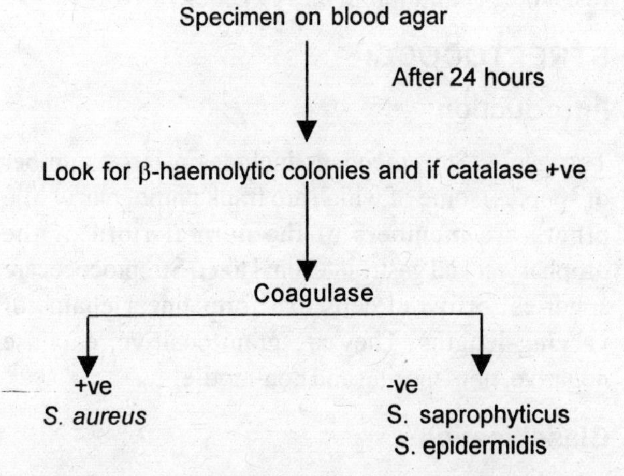


| *Characteristic* | *S. aureus* | *S. epidermidis* | *S. saprophyticus* |
|---|---|---|---|
| Colour of colonies | Yellow to white | White | White to pale grey |
| Haemolysis | + | ± | - |
| Coagulase production | Yes | No | No |
| Mannitol fermentation | Yes | No | Yes |
| Novobiocin sensitivity | Sensitive | Sensitive | Resistant |

## Other Media for Isolation of Staphylococci

- Milk agar to enhance pigment
- Phenolphthalein phosphate agar.
- Selective salt media.
- Mannitol salt agar.

### *Treatment*

**Benzyl penicillin** is effective if strain is sensitive. In case of penicillin resistance, **Methicillin, Oxacillin, Nafcillin** or **first generation cephalosporins** are given.

**Vancomycin** is the drug of choice for Methicillin resistant *S. aureus* (MRSA). MRSA is resistant to most of commonly used antibiotics. Mupirocin is used to remove carriage. MRSA is chromosomal resistance (mutation in *mec* A gene).

# STREPTOCOCCI

## Introduction

The genus *Streptococcus* includes a large number of species, some of which are frank pathogens, while others are members of the normal flora of the oropharynx and gastrointestinal tract. Streptococci are spherical or ovoid cells that form linear chains of varying lengths. They are gram-positive, catalase negative, non-sporing and non-motile.

## Classification

A. The first system of classification is based on the type of **haemolysis**.

1. **$\alpha$-haemolytic streptococci- incomplete haemolysis**- which imparts green appearance to the haemoglobin.
2. **$\beta$-haemolytic streptococci-complete haemolysis**- clear zone in the agar. *S. pyogenes* is the most important pathogen.
3. **$\gamma$-haemolytic streptococci- non-haemolytic.**

B. **Lancefield system**

This classification is based upon the grouping of the streptococcal **cell wall carbohydrate called the C antigen**—divided into serologic groups from A to W, (with the exception of I and J). Group A β-haemolytic streptococci, that cause many human infections, are given the species name *Streptococcus pyogenes.* Other groups that have serious human pathogens include B, C, D and G.

The species can be grouped on the basis of antigenic differences of cell wall proteins (e.g. M, T and R proteins).

C. **Phylogenetic relationship**

On the basis of 16S rRNA sequence of members of the genus, it has been divided into 6 clusters:

1. **Pyogenic group**—consists of β-haemolytic species, pathogenic to humans.
2. **Anginosus group**—found in oral, gastro-intestinal and genital tract.
3. **Mitis group**—includes *Streptococcus pneumoniae* and several oral streptococci.
4. **Salivarius group**—includes dairy streptococci and species in human oral cavity.
5. **Bovis group**—organisms in the intestinal canal of several animal species.
6. **Mutans group**—organisms that colonise the tooth surface of humans.

**Group A β-haemolytic *S. pyogenes***

– most important human pathogen amongst streptococci.

## Antigenic Structure

- The cell wall of streptococci consists of an outer layer of protein, a middle layer of group-specific carbohydrate and an inner layer of peptidoglycan.
- Group specific carbohydrate- it can be extracted by a number of methods as HCl (**Lancefield acid extraction**), formamide **(Fuller's method)**, enzyme produced by *Streptomyces albus*

**(Maxted's method)** and autoclaving **(Rantz & Randall method).**

- Proteins- *S. pyogenes* produces 3 surface protein antigens-(M,T & R), which help in serological typing.
- **M protein** is the most important as it acts as a virulence factor by inhibiting phagocytosis. It is acid and heat stable while trypsin sensitive. Typing is done by **capillary precipitation** method.
- **T protein** is resistant to pepsin and trypsin but heat and acid stable. Typing is done by **slide agglutination** method.
- **R protein** is destroyed by pepsin but not by trypsin.

Determinants of pathogenicity and virulence

| *Factors* | *Major biological activities* |
|---|---|
| **Proteins** | |
| M protein | Have antiphagocytic and anticomplement properties. |
| Protein F (fibronectin binding protein) | Adhesion factor that along with Protein M enables Group A streptococci to bind to pharyngeal epithelial cells. |
| Protein G<br>Adhesion factor. | Binds IgG through wrong site (i.e. Fc portion) to inhibit phagocytosis. |
| **Erythrogenic toxins** | |
| **Streptococcal Pyrogenic Exotoxins** | Are closely related to staphylococcal enterotoxins. |
| SPE A | It is a **superantigen** responsible for systemic manifestations of Group streptococcal infections. |
| SPE B | It is a cysteine protease that causes tissue destruction in necrotizing fasciitis. |
| SPE C | It is also a **superantigen** with biological effects similar to SPE A. |
| **Streptolysins** | |
| Streptolysin O (oxygen labile) | It causes lysis of RBC's.<br>Plays role in development of Rheumatic Fever.<br>It is highly immunogenic and induces the production of **antistreptolysin O (ASLO) antibodies** which can be demonstrated within 10-14 days. It is an indicator of prior or recent streptococcal infection. |

*Contd.*

*Contd.*

| | |
|---|---|
| Streptolysin S (serum soluble) | It causes β-haemolysis of colonies of most pyogenic streptococci on aerobically incubated blood agar. It is non-immunogenic. |
| **Spreading factors** Streptokinase (fibrinolysin) | Binds to human plasminogen to form protease plasmin that cleaves fibrin and fibrinogen- thereby, causing spread of infection by lysing the clot. |
| Streptodornase (deoxyribonucleases) | Depolymerizes DNA in thick pus to spread infection. |
| C5a peptidase | Inhibits opsonization. |
| Hyaluronidase | Cleaves intercellular hyaluronic acid to spread infection. |
| Nucleases (DNAases A-D) | DNA ase B is predominant in *S. pyogenes*. |
| Neuraminidases | Helps in invasion. |
| NAD ases | Its role in virulence is unclear. Antibodies to it may be formed during infection. |
| Serum opacity factor (SOF) lipoproteinase | Produced by Group A *Streptococcus* of certain M types. Help in M typing. |

## Non-suppurative Sequelae

- **Acute rheumatic fever**: pathogenesis is not completely understood. Theories to focus on the tissue damage caused by streptococcal products (i.e. streptolysins) or antigen-antibody complexes. More recent theories incorporate the concepts of molecular mimicry and autoimmunity. Antibodies directed against streptococcal products are thought to cross-react with host tissue producing autoimmune damage.
- **Acute poststreptococcal glomerulonephritis**: deposition of immune complexes on the epithelial side of the glomerular basement membrane cause an inflammatory response. The concept of molecular mimicry is also illustrated by cross-reaction with human glomeruli of antibodies raised against streptococcal membrane components.

Structural components of *Streptococcus pyogenes* which cross-react with human tissues

| *Strept pyogenes* structural components | Human tissue with which it cross-reacts |
|---|---|
| Capsular hyaluronic acid | Synovial fluid |
| Cell wall protein | Myocardium |
| Cell wall carbohydrate | Cardiac valves |
| Cytoplasmic membrane | Vascular intima |
| peptidoglycan | Skin |

## Clinical Disease

Primary infections of group A streptococci are generally **suppurative** (i.e. characterised by pus formation). **Nonsuppurative** sequelae may follow primary infection by group A streptococci and presumably result from cross-reactive autoimmunity triggered by the host's response to the microbe or tissue damage inflicted by streptococcal toxins and extracellular factors. Attempt to isolate the organism is usually unsuccessful.

| *Primary infection* | *Type of infection* | *Clinical presentation* |
|---|---|---|
| **Suppurative** | Pharyngitis | Most common bacterial impetigo cause of (viruses are more common). Fever malaise, headache and sore throat. |
| | Pyoderma and pharyngitis | It is characterised by superficial skin infections. |
| | Erysipelas | It is the spreading infection of skin and mucous or mucous membranes, usually on the face. |
| | Cellulitis | Inflammation of the skin and underlying connective tissue. |
| | Puerperal fever | Infection of the uterus following childbirth. |
| | Necrotizing fascitis | Invasive soft tissue infection characterised by extensive fascial and subcutaneous tissue necrosis. |
| | Otitis media, sinusitis, mastoiditis, | |

*Contd.*

*Contd.*

| | | |
|---|---|---|
| | bacteraemia and pneumonia | |
| **Toxin mediated** Erythrogenic toxin | Scarlet fever | Fever with papular red rash over the whole body, blanches on pressure and peeling of skin after fever subsides. |
| Pyrogenic exotoxin A | Streptococcal toxic shock syndrome | Similar to toxic shock syndrome induced by staphylococcal toxins. |
| **Non-suppurative sequelae** | Rheumatic fever | Follows streptococcal throat infection and diagnosis is based upon the Jones criteria and serological evidence of a previous streptococcal infection (an elevated levels of ASLO and anti-DNAase antibodies). |
| | Acute poststrepto-coccal glomerulo-nephritis | It usually follows cutaneous infections, and may also follow pharyngeal infections. |

## Epidemiology

Group A streptococci causing pharyngitis and respiratory infections are usually transmitted from patient to patient via respiratory or saliva droplets. Respiratory carriage rate in healthy school going children is higher (15-20%) than adults.

The primary skin infections are initiated by streptococci colonizing the intact skin, while the secondary infections of traumatized skin include those of surgical wounds and burns.

Since the development of ARF and AGN is directly linked to antecedent streptococcal infections, the epidemiology of most cases of these diseases is similar to that of streptococcal pharyngitis. The variables are mentioned as rheumatogenic or nephritogenic strains. Proper treatment of streptococcal pharyngitis can decrease the incidence of rheumatic fever.

## Laboratory Diagnosis

**Suppurative infections:** Diagnosis is based upon the identification of β-haemolytic streptococci isolated.

**Microscopy**: On direct examination of a Gram stain of the specimen gram-positive cocci in chains is diagnostic.

**Culture:** The specimen can be plated on blood agar for isolation of streptococci. The media is inoculated and incubated at 37° C for 24 hours.

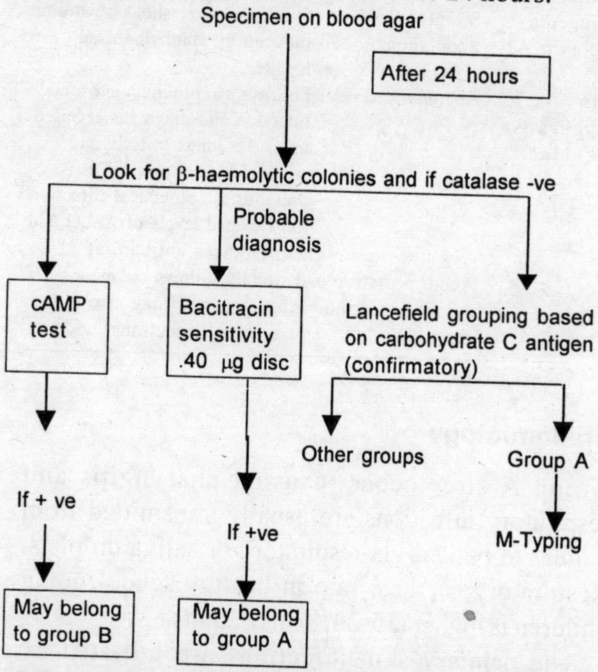


**Other media**: Pike's media (blood agar containing crystal violet and sodium azide) is used as a transport media in case of a delay.

**Columbia blood agar, PNF media** and **Crystal Violet Blood Agar** are the other selective media used for isolation of streptococci.

**Non-suppurative sequelae:** Diagnosis is based upon demonstration of increased titre of antibodies to one or more streptococcal antigens.

A retrospective diagnosis of streptococcal infection may be established by serology in ARF and AGN. The most commonly used test is the **ASLO test** in which titres higher than 200 Todd units/ml is indicative of prior streptococcal infection. The other test is the

**ADNase** in which titres higher than 300 or 350 are significant.

### Treatment

**Penicillin** is the effective drug of choice and no resistance has yet been observed. In patients allergic to penicillin, erythromycin or cephalosporins are the alternatives.

## Group B Streptococci

Group B streptococci were earlier associated as the pathogens for cattle, but in 1930's their association with human diseases was discovered. Group B streptococci are found in the genital tract of 5-50% pregnant women. The infections that they cause are:

**Neonatal Infections**

**Early onset-** occurs within the first few days of life. It manifests in preterm infants or those whose mothers exhibited obstructive complications. The neonate exhibits symptoms of lethargy, poor feeding, fever and respiratory symptoms, and develops bacteraemia and pneumonia within the first week of infection. These infections are associated with a high mortality rate of 0-70%.

**Late onset-** begins within 1 week to 3 months of age. The baby acquires infection from the hospital and not the mother. There is no bacteraemia or meningitis and it's associated with a more favourable outcome, though neurological sequelae are more common.

**Adult infections**

Postpartum infections are the most common. Other infections include septicaemia, skin and soft tissue infections, endocarditis, meningitis, genital and urinary tract infections.

**Laboratory Diagnosis**

On blood agar, group B streptococci produce α-haemolysis. In addition, hydrolysis of sodium hippurate and **CAMP** test (Christie Atkins Munch-Peterson) are the tests for presumptive diagnosis. Lancefield grouping is the confirmatory test.

### Treatment

Ampicillin is the drug of choice.

### Infection by Group C and G Streptococci

These are normal commensals of the respiratory tract, intestinal tract, skin and genital tract. They are of two types, which include large colony formers and small colony forming strains belonging to *Streptococcus milleri* group. These organisms are associated with wide infections as sore throat, skin and wound infections, endocarditis, meningitis and bone infections.

### Group D Streptococci

These can be divided into enterococci and non-enterococci.

Enteroccoci were considered a part of streptococci earlier but based on G + C content they have been separated into separate genus *Enterococcus.*

They have the ability to grow in the presence of 40% bile and hydrolyze aesculin. They are normal flora in the lower intestinal tract and vagina.

### Enterococci

- Species most commonly associated with human infections are *E. faecalis* and *E. faecium.*
- They grow on blood agar, 6.5% sodium chloride, 40% bile and pH 9.6.
- On MacConkey medium, they give pink colonies.
- They may be β-haemolytic, α-haemolytic or non-haemolytic on blood agar.
- The infections caused by enterococci include UTI, infective endocarditis, biliary tract infections, peritonitis, suppurative abdominal lesions and septicaemia.

- These are associated with drug resistance problems and most of the strains are resistant to penicillin and sulphonamides. Some are even vancomycin resistant.

**Non-enterococci Group D streptococci**- the common organisms are S.b*ovis, S. equinum* and *S. avium,* they do not grow in 6.5% sodium chloride and are susceptible to penicillin. They cause infections as UTI, endocarditis and septicaemia.

## Viridans Streptococci

- These organisms commonly inhabit the oral cavity and upper respiratory tract. These organisms lack the overt virulence factors of pyogenic group; yet can participate in a variety of infections.
- The members include *S. salivarius, S. sanguis, S. mutans* and *S. mitis.*
- They have been associated with dental caries and in persons with predisposing factors as vascular disease of the heart, may cause **infective endocarditis**, especially after dental manipulations, which lead to their entry into the bloodstream following injury of the oral canal. This leads to **transient bacteraemia**, creating favourable conditions for colonization of heart valves. They are also associated with dental caries.

## Streptococcus Pneumoniae

- *Streptococcus pneumoniae* are gram-positive, catalase negative cocci, which are ovoid, or **lancet-shaped** and often seen in pairs (**diplococci**).
- They are non-sporing and non-motile.
- The organisms are **capsulated** and the capsule can be best seen in specimen collected directly from the exudates.
- They grow best under increased carbon dioxide tension (5-10%), which can be obtained in a candle jar (**capnophilic** organisms).

## Classification

Pneumococci are divided into 90 serotypes on the basis of capsular polysaccharide, named 1, 2, 3... Since it lacks group specific cell wall antigens, pneumococci cannot be classified using the Lancefield system of classification.

## Antigenic Structure and Virulence

### *Capsule*

- The pneumococcal polysaccharide capsule is essential for virulence, protecting the organism from phagocytosis.
- The capsular polysaccharide antigen is also the basis of serotyping.
- Only the smooth S strain is pathogenic to man. The capsule can be demonstrated by **Quellung reaction**.
- The antibodies to capsular polysaccharide are protective and a basis of many polysaccharide vaccines for immunization.

**C polysaccharide (C substance)**-composed of techoic acid and peptidoglycan.

**F antigen**-can evoke heterophile antibodies that cross-react with antigens of Forssman series.

**C-reactive proteins**-abnormal proteins (α-globulin). It appears in acute phase of severe pneumonia. It is known as C reactive protein as it precipitates with C antigen of pneumococci.

**IgA1 protease**-cleaves IgA1 which leads to reduction in phagocytosis.

**Autolysin and pneumolysin**-autolysin leads to activation of intracellular pneumolysin which further causes decreased neutrophil chemotaxis, phagocytosis and immune responses.

**Others**-pneumococcal surface protein **PspA** (similar to M protein of *S. pyogenes*), neuraminidase, hyaluronidase and other proteolytic enzymes.

## Clinical Disease

Pneumococcal pneumonia is rarely a primary infection and results when normal defence barriers of respiratory tract are disturbed. The **bacterial pneumonia** is common in children and adults. Other infections include—otitis media, meningitis, sinusitis, bronchitis, endocarditis, suppurative arthritis and peritonitis.

### Predisposing Factors

- Conditions that cause impaired immune responses.
- Viral induced immunosuppression.
- Loss of splenic function.

### Laboratory Diagnosis

### Direct Demonstration

Pneumococci can be directly demonstrated in samples as sputum, CSF, blood and exudates. On Gram stain, they are seen as gram-positive diplococci usually surrounded by a capsule.

The pneumococcal antigen can be demonstrated directly by Latex agglutination and coagglutination.

### Culture

Pneumococci can be isolated by plating the specimen onto blood agar and chocolate agar in the presence of 5-10% $CO_2$ and incubating at 37° C for 18-24 hours. The colonies that appear are α-haemolytic which on further incubation develop a central depression due to autolysis (**draughtsman colonies**). These colonies are catalase negative, show **bile solubility** and **sensitivity to optochin** (0.5 μg disc and a zone size >14 mm).

### Serotyping

It is done based on the capsular polysaccharide antigen typing.

### Quellung Reaction

It is based on the interaction of capsular polysaccharide and the corresponding antibody. This causes changes in the optical properties of the capsule, causing it to **appear swollen** (appears more refractile) when observed under the microscope.

### Confirmation of Diagnosis

It is done by intraperitoneal inoculation in mice—leads to its death in 1-3 days. Pneumococci can be isolated in peritoneal exudates, heart and blood on postmortem examination.

### Treatment

Penicillin is the drug of choice, but resistant strains have been isolated due to **chromosomally mediated** changes in penicillin binding proteins (PBP) in cell wall. Cephalosporins are the alternative drugs. Vancomycin with or without rifampicin is given in highly resistant strains.

### Control and Prevention

**Polyvalent vaccine** made from capsular polysaccharide of 23 serological groups is recommended for high-risk individuals.

## GRAM-POSITIVE RODS (BACILLI)

The gram-positive rods can be classified as either non-spore forming or spore-forming. *Bacillus* and *Clostridium* form spores, whereas *Corynebacterium* and *Listeria* do not. Members of the genus *Bacillus* are aerobic, whereas those of the genus *Clostridium* are anaerobic.

## CORYNEBACTERIA

The coryneform bacteria are pleomorphic, gram-positive, non-motile, catalase positive bacilli that are members of the normal flora of the skin, nasopharynx, oropharynx, urogenital tract and gastrointestinal tract. These species are collectively known as **diphtheroids.**

The major pathogen is *C. diphtheriae.*

## Classification

Most corynebacteria are nutritionally exacting except the lipophilic ones, whose growth is stimulated by lipids as Tween 80, oleic acid, egg yolk or serum. Hence, they are divided into two groups:

| *Lipophilic **Corynebacterium spp.*** | *Nonlipophilic Corynebacterium **spp.*** |
|---|---|
| *C. diphtheriae* | *C. xerosis* |
| *C. ulcerans* | *C. minutissimum* |
| *C. pseudotuberculosis* | *C. striatum* |
| *C. jeikeium* | *C. pseudodiphtheriticum* |
| *C. urealyticum* | |

The ***Corynebacterium diphtheriae*** **group:**

Members of this group include ***C. diphtheriae, C. ulcerans*** and ***C. pseudotuberculosis.***

These organisms are separated from other corynebacteria by their ability to **form exotoxin, lack of pyrizinamidase and presence of palmitoleic acid.**

### *Corynebacterium diphtheriae*

They are gram-positive pleomorphic rods with clubbed ends (coryne means club), non-capsulated, non-motile and are arranged in angled pairs or parallel rows, resembling **Chinese letters**, also known as **cuneiform arrangement.**

## Granules

- The organisms may also contain granules of polyphosphates which act as storage depots. They stain metachromatically (meaning different colour) with methylene blue or toluidine blue. The granules take up a reddish-purplish colour and are known as **metachromatic** or **Babes-Ernst** or **volutin granules or polymetaphosphate granules**.
- With **Albert stain**, the granules take up a bluish black stain and the cytoplasm is green.
- Due to the presence of granules, the organism stains unevenly on **Gram staining** giving it a **granular appearance**.

- The presence of granules differentiates *C. diphtheriae* from the other non-pathogenic diphtheroids.

> Diphtheroids stain more uniformly than diphtheria bacilli, are arranged in palisades rather than Chinese letter arrangement and possess no granules.

## Growth Characters

It grows well on blood agar but growth is improved in **Loeffler's agar** (grows fast on it and colonies appear in 6-8 hours) and **potassium tellurite containing blood agar (Tinsdale or Hoyle's medium).**
On the basis of growth on blood tellurite agar medium, diphtheria bacilli can be divided into four biotypes: mitis, intermedius, gravis and belfanti.

Differentiation of the biotypes of *C. diphtheriae*

| *Character* | *Gravis* | *Intermedius* | *Mitis* |
|---|---|---|---|
| Morphology | Short, stain uniformly, less pleomorphic, few granules | Long, highly pleomorphic, poor granulation | Long, pleomorphic, granulated |
| Colony characters on blood tellurite agar | **Daisy head** colony | **Frog's egg** colony | **Poached egg** colony |
| Haemolysis | Weakly haemolytic | Non-haemolytic | β-haemolytic |
| Starch and glycogen reduction | + | – | – |
| Toxigenicity | Almost 100% | 95-99% | 80-85% |
| Predominant strains | Epidemic areas | Epidemic areas | Endemic areas |

* *C. diphtheriae* subsp.b*elfanti* has been derived from biotype mitis except that it does not reduce nitrate to nitrite unlike the other biotypes.

## Pathogenicity

*C. diphtheriae* is not an invasive organism; systemic symptom[illegible] [illegible]uction of an **exotoxin** [illegible] do not cause systemic dise[illegible]

Only those strains of C. *diphtheriae* that have been lysogenized by a β-phage carrying the *tox* gene produce diphtheria toxin. Non-toxigenic strains can be rendered toxigenic by infecting them with β-phage. This is known as **lysogenic or phage conversion.**

Toxin synthesis is regulated by the availability of iron, peaks at a low concentration of 0.1 mg per litre of the medium and stops at 0.5 mg per litre of the medium.

## Mechanism of Action

The exotoxin is a protein with two components:

**Fraction B**—for attachment to the cells and transport into the cell.

**Fraction A**—it is the active moiety and is responsible for the biological properties of the toxin. It acts by **inhibition of polypeptide chain elongation** by causing ribosylation of EF-2.

## Epidemiology

*C. diphtheriae* is transmitted by direct contact or respiratory droplets.

Children are most commonly infected.

## Clinical Disease

### Local effect

When the toxigenic bacteria get lodged in the oropharynx by attachment to the receptor, they multiply and produce the exotoxin leading to local tissue necrosis. The combination of necrotic material and inflammatory exudates leads to the formation of a **pseudomembrane** over the **tonsils, uvula, soft palate or pharyngeal wall**.

The pseudomembrane spreads upward into the **nasal passage** and downward into the **larynx** and **trachea**, causing mechanical obstruction leading to suffocation unless the airway obstruction is restored.

The most common **cause of death** is due to suffocation due to **airway obstruction**.

**Systemic effect**

The diphtheria bacilli **do not penetrate the deep underlying tissue** but the exotoxin **gets absorbed into the bloodstream** leading to systemic complications. There is no bacteremia but there is toxemia.

The toxin has a special affinity for heart muscles, peripheral nerves and adrenal glands.

The most common complication leading to death is **myocarditis.**

## Diagnosis

The initial diagnosis is based upon clinical presentation.

Specific treatment (antitoxin) should be initiated immediately without waiting for lab confirmation.

Diagnosis is based upon culture and isolation of toxin producing *C. diphtheriae (CD).*

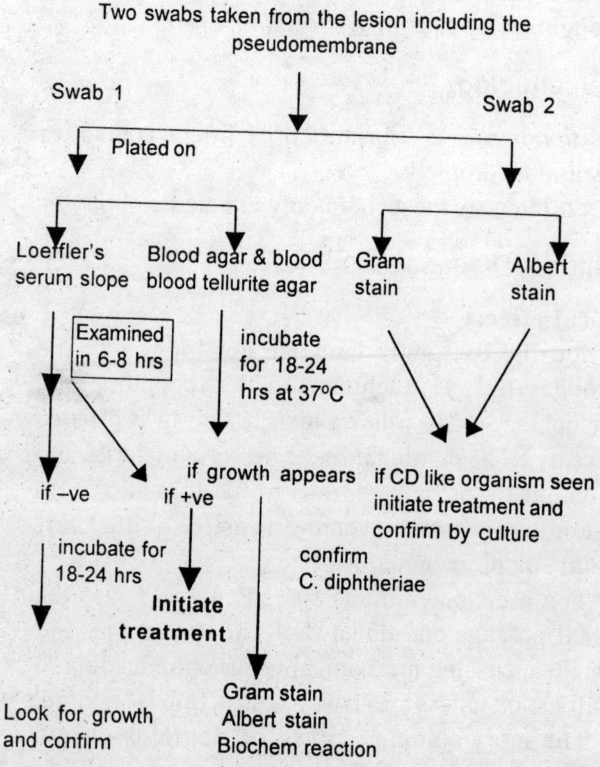

## Toxigenicity Testing

Once identified, diphtheria bacilli should be promptly tested for toxigenicity. These tests are of two types:

### *A. In Vivo*

1. **Subcutaneous test:** Colonies of *Corynebacterium diphtheriae* are inoculated subcutaneously into 2 guinea pigs. One of them is protected with intraperitoneal inoculation of 1000 units of antitoxin 3 hrs prior to the test while the other is unprotected. If the organism is *Corynebacterium diphtheriae* then the unprotected animal dies within 96 hours. **The autopsy findings reveal:**
   - Gelatinous haemorrhagic oedema at the site of inoculation.
   - Haemorrhagic pleural and peritoneal exudate.
   - Haemorrhagic inflammation of the adrenal glands.
     - If both the animals die—strain is toxigenic but not *C. diphtheriae.*
     - If **neither animal dies—it is non-toxigenic.**
2. **Intradermal test:** After inoculating the culture intradermally in the guinea pig, it is given 500 units of antitoxin intraperitoneally after four hours. Non-specific inflammation is seen within 24-48 hours, and if the strain is toxigenic, the site where the test dose was inoculated will progress to necrotic lesion in 48-72 hours. Hence, the animal does not die in this test.

### *B. In Vitro*

**Elek's gel precipitation test:** It is a double-diffusion test performed directly on the surface of an agar late. A filter paper strip is impregnated with antiserum and incorporated to the agar medium. The test strain is streaked at right angle to the antitoxin strip. If the strain is toxin producing, precipitin lines of the toxin with the antitoxin will appear.

## Treatment

The treatment should entail neutralization of the toxin, antibiotic therapy and supportive measures.

**Diphtheria antitoxin** in doses proportional to the severity of the infection (20,000-100,000 units) is administered promptly.

**Penicillin** is the antibiotic of choice and is given to kill the diphtheria bacilli present in the throat and prevent toxin production.

**Supportive measures** include tracheostomy for airway obstruction and CVS support for myocarditis.

## Prevention and Control

The methods of immunization include:

1. **Active immunization** with DPT vaccine, which consists of diphtheria toxoid in combination with tetanus toxoid and killed suspension of pertussis bacilli. It is given at the age of 6, 10 and 14 weeks and 16-24 months followed by a booster of DT at 5-6 years.
2. **Passive immunization:** during emergency, 500-1000 units of antidiphtheritic serum (ADS) is administered subcutaneously, when the susceptible individuals are exposed to the infection.
3. **Combined immunization:** ADS is administered on one arm and first dose active immunization on the other.

Non-diphtheria *Corynebacterium*

| *Organism* | *Spectrum of disease and infection* |
|---|---|
| *C. ulcerans* | Associated with diphtheria like sore throat. |
| *C. pseudotuberculosis* | Suppurative granulomatous lymphadenitis. |
| *C. jeikeium* | Septicaemia, wound infection and endocarditis in immunocompromised patients, especially those with intravenous catheters. |
| *C. pseudo-diptheriticum* | Endocarditis and pneumonia in immunosuppressed. |
| *C. minutissimum* | Superficial pruritic skin infections known as erythrasma. |
| *C. urealyticum* | UTI and skin infections in immunocompromised patients. |
| *C. xerosis* | Endocarditis and septicaemia in immunocompromised individuals. |

## LISTERIA

It is widely distributed in nature and behaves as an opportunistic agent in humans. It consists of gram-positive, motile rods, is catalase positive and grows on the common media as sheep blood agar to produce β-haemolytic colonies.

*Listeria monocytogenes,* an intracellular parasite, produces infection in the very young and in immunocompromised adults.

**Neonatal listeriosis** is characterized by **meningitis** during the first three weeks of life while **adult listeriosis** may present from mild influenza like syndrome to fulminant listeriosis. The most common infection is **meningitis**. It can also cause **bacteraemia** and **endocarditis**.

## BACILLUS

The genus *Bacillus* comprises aerobes and facultative anaerobic, gram-positive bacilli, which are **characterised by spore formation**. It comprises of more than 40 species, of which only two: *B. anthracis* and *B. cereus* cause human and animal diseases.

**Historical importance of genus *Bacillus***

- Koch demonstrated the Koch's postulates in studies on anthrax.
- Pasteur developed the first bacteria vaccine against anthrax.
- *B. anthracis* was the first pathogenic bacterium to be observed under the microscope.
- Koch and Pasteur demonstrated the germ theory of disease with *B. anthracis.*

**Practical applications of genus Bacillus in research field**

- *B. stearothermophilus or B. subtilis* incorporated in filter paper strips are used as controls in thermal sterilization procedures.
- *B. thuringiensis* is used as an insecticide or pest control on food crops **(Biological control of vectors).**

- *B.subtilis* provides a model for microbial genetics.
- They serve as a source of various antibiotics as bacitracin (*B. licheniformis* or *B. subtilis)* and polymixin (*B. polymyxa*).

## B. anthracis

It consists of gram-positive, nonmotile, spore forming bacilli.

- In smears obtained from infected tissues, they are surrounded by a capsule, which is **polypeptide** in nature unlike other bacteria which have polysaccharide capsule. The capsule can be demonstrated by staining blood films containing anthrax with polychrome methylene blue. On examination under the microscope, the capsule appears as amorphous purplish material around the bacilli—known as **McFadyean's reaction.**
- The spores are formed in unfavourable conditions, are oval and central (giving the organism **box-car appearance** on staining).
- The ends of the bacilli are swollen so that chain of bacilli presents a **bamboo-stick** appearance.

## Cultural Characteristics

- When the growth of the bacteria on nutrient agar medium is examined under the microscope, the edge of the colony is found to be composed of long, interlacing chains of bacteria resembling curled hair-lock. This gives them the **medusa head** appearance.
- A selective medium known as **PLET medium** (consisting of heart infusion agar with polymyxin, lysozyme, EDTA and thallous acetate) is used to isolate *B. anthracis.*
- In a gelatine stab culture, the growth is down the stab line giving an **inverted fir tree** appearance.

The pathogenicity is determined by the **capsule** and an **exotoxin** that consists of three protein components-protective antigen (PA), lethal factor (LA) and edema factor (EF).

## Clinical Disease

Anthrax is a zoonosis, a disease of animals transmissible to man. Man acquires infection through small cuts and abrasions, inhalation or ingestion. The disease may manifest as:

**Cutaneous anthrax:** It is the most common clinical presentation and is also know as **malignant pustule**. It is common in farmers, veterinary doctors and animal or animal product handlers. The lesion starts as a small, painless papule which develops into a vesicle and then ruptures releasing a dark fluid and leading to an eschar surrounded by inflammation.

**Pulmonary anthrax:** It is also known as **wool sorter's disease**, acquired by inhalation of spores from infected wool. It is a haemorrhagic pneumonia that can be fatal.

**Gastrointestinal anthrax:** It occurs due to ingestion of contaminated food leading to haemorrhagic diarrhoea.

**Others**: Bacteraemia or secondary infections as meningitis can occur as complications.

The drug of choice for treatment is **Penicillin.**

A live attenuated spore vaccine made from a noncapsulated strain of *B. anthracis* is used for animal vaccine. No human vaccine is available.

## Bacillus Cereus

It is widely distributed in the environment and may cause human disease, especially in immuocompromised individuals.

It is aerobic,spore-forming gram-positive bacilli resembling *B. anthracis* except that it **is motile and lacks the glutamic acid capsule.**

It produces 2 toxins—**emetic toxin** (associated with food poisoning) and **enterotoxin** (associated with diarrhoeal syndrome).

### Food poisoning

*Bacillus cereus* causes food poisoning, which occurs 1-6 hours after the consumption of food contaminated with the emetic toxin (boiled or **fried rice** is a common source). *Bacillus cereus* spores may germinate in the food and release the enterotoxin, which leads to adenyl cyclase activation causing an increased level of cAMP that causes profuse diarrhoea. Patient usually recovers 6-24 hours after the onset of symptoms.

An enormous number of organisms ($10^5$ or more per gram of are found in the contaminated food). Since the infection is self-limiting, only supportive treatment is required.

*B. cereus* can cause systemic infections in immunocompromised patients. The treatment of choice in such cases is **clindamycin.**

### *B. subtilis*

It causes infection in immunocompromised individuals as in intravenous drug users, leading to septicaemia. Penicillin is the drug of choice.

## CLOSTRIDIUM

- These organisms are **anaerobic**, gram-positive spore bearing bacilli.
- They are motile except ***C. perfringens.***
- The spores are wider than the vegetative forms, giving them a bulging spindle shape.
- In 1861, Pasteur discovered anaerobiosis and the first discovered anaerobe was *C. butyricum.*
- Clostridia lack the **catalase, peroxidases and superoxide dismutase** that are responsible for destroying the toxic radicals produced in the presence of oxygen; hence they grow only in anaerobic conditions.
- Clostridia are widely distributed in nature, but their principal habitats are soil and intestinal tract of animals.

### Classification

*Clostridium* can be divided on the basis of biochemical tests into:

1. Predominantly saccharolytic clostridia:
   - *C. perfringens*
   - *C. septicum*
   - *C. fallax*
2. Predominately proteolytic clostridia
   - *C. sporogenes*
   - *C. histolyticum*
3. Slightly proteolytic clostridia
   - *C. tetani*

**Saccharolytic-** when grown in cooked meat broth; the organisms produce acid and gas but do not digest the meat. The meat is reddened.
**Proteolytic**-they digest meat and liquefy gelatin. Culture in cooked meat broth produces blackening of the meat.

### *Clostridium perfringens (C. welchii)*

- They are gram-positive, non-motile and spore-bearing (subterminal or central) organisms.
- Spores are rarely seen in direct smears from specimen, but can be induced in a special medium known as the **Ellner's medium.**
- In litmus milk, it ferments lactose and produces acid and gas. The acid clots the mil and gas breaks the clot resulting in **stormy reaction.**
- Gelatine is liquefied and it is saccharolytic.

## Virulence and Toxigenicity

*Clostridium perfringens* produces 12 exotoxins (4 major lethal and 8 minor) and an enterotoxin. On the basis of 4 major toxins, *C. perfringens* can be divided into 5 types, A to E

**(A) Exotoxins**

The major exotoxins are:

**α (alpha), β (beta), ε(epsilon)** and **ι(iota).**

**α-toxin**—It is produced by all types, but most abundantly by A strains.

It is $Ca^{++}$ or $Mg^{++}$ dependant phospholipase (a **lecithinase)** and the most important toxin that is responsible for the toxaemia of gas gangrene.

It produces opalescence in serum or egg-yolk containing media by splitting phospholipids complexes. This reaction can be inhibited by specific antitoxin—a basis of **Naegler's reaction.**

*C. perfringens* is the most common cause of gas gangrene (60-80%) and most common toxin type of the organism assumed is type A.

The minor lethal toxins include:

γ (gamma), δ (delta), κ (kappa), λ (lambda), μ (mu), η (nu), θ (theta) and ν (eta).

## (B). Enterotoxin

It is produced by *Clostridium perfringens* type A strain and is produced in the intestine during the time of sporulation. It inhibits glucose transport, causes protein loss and epithelial damage.

Pathogenesis and clinical disease

| *Infection caused* | *Pathogenesis* | *Clinical presentation* |
|---|---|---|
| **Gas gangrene** | | |
| Most common cause (60-80%) and mostly by toxin type A. | It develops due to **reduced oxidation-reduction** potential. Failure of blood supply due to trauma, presence of foreign bodies, casts or dressings, haemorrhage in the wound, etc. lead to germination of spores. | **Wound contamination-** presence of clostridium in the traumatized tissue. **Clostridial cellulites-** infection confined to the tissues in the absence of toxaemia. **Clostridial myonecrosis or gas gangrene-** invasion of muscles and toxaemia. There is increased pain, tenderness, oedema of the affected part with signs of systemic toxaemia. |
| **Food poisoning** | Due to enterotoxin **production in the intestine**. It inserts and disrupts membranes of the mucosal cells. | Abdominal cramps, diarrhoea and vomiting occur within 8-12 hours of ingestion of contaminated food and subside by 24 hours. |
| Necrotic enteritis | A severe and often fatal condition caused by β-toxin of *C. perfringens* type C. | Acute abdominal pain, bloody diarrhoea, ulceration and perforation of the intestine and toxaemia. |

## Diagnosis

- The diagnosis of gas gangrene should be made on clinical grounds.
- The role of the lab comes in the confirmation of the clinical diagnosis.
- Presence of gram-positive, thick, stubby rods with other bacilli can be confirmed by aerobic and anaerobic cultures on blood agar.
- For isolation from faeces in case of food poisoning, sample is inoculated on cooked meat broth. A count $\sim 10^6$ bacteria/g of faeces material is characteristic of food poisoning.
- Subculture on Willis and Hobb's medium and looking for Nagler's reaction are some of the other tests.

## Prophylaxis and Treatment

*Gas Gangrene*

- **Wound debridement** and irrigation of the wound to remove clots, foreign material and necrotic tissue is the most important.
- **Hyperbaric oxygen** is also recommended to stop the growth of the organism and release of the toxin.
- Antimicrobial therapy help accelerate recovery. **Penicillin** is the drug of choice.
- **Antitoxic therapy** with polyvalent antisera is also used.

*Food Poisoning*

Treatment is essentially supportive.

*Clostridium tetani*

- These are gram-positive pleomorphic bacilli, are non-capsulated and **motile** by a peritrichate flagella.
- They possess terminal spores that give them a **drumstick appearance.**
- It grows well on cooked meat broth and blood agar on which it shows β-haemolysis (due to production of tetanolysin).

- It is slightly proteolytic and liquefies gelatine slowly.

### Virulence and Toxigenicity

*C. tetani* produces two biologically active agents: the **neurotoxin** or **tetanospasmin** and an oxygen labile haemolysin known as **tetanolysin**.

### Tetanospasmin

It is a powerful toxin that is plasmid encoded. It acts by blocking the inhibitory pathways in the CNS resulting in spasticity and convulsions. The neurotransmitter for these pathways is **γ-aminobutyric acid (GABA).**

**Tetanolysin:** It is antigenically related to streptolysin O and θ-toxin of *C. perfringens* and *C. novyi.* Their role in disease pathogenesis is not yet known.

### Pathogenicity

Tetanus develops following the contamination of wound by *C. tetani* spores. The organism establishes a localized infection and elaborates the potent tetanospasmin, which mediates generalized muscle spasms.

Conditions that favour spore germination and progression of symptoms are similar to those of C. *perfringens.*

The toxin is absorbed from the site of production and ascends to the CNS via the peripheral nerve endings.

### Clinical Disease

The incubation period varies from few days to several weeks. The types include:

**Localized tetanus:** there is persistent spasm around the injury site. This is a mild form.

**Cephalic tetanus:** associated with dysfunction of one or more cranial nerves.

**Generalized tetanus:** most common form, characterized by spasm of potent muscles.

**Tetanus neonatorum** and **uterine tetanus** has a high fatality in India.

**Diagnosis**

- The diagnosis is usually based on clinical findings.
- *C. tetani* can be isolated on blood agar and CMB from wound scrapings and debrided tissue. On blood agar, the colonies exhibit a dentate spreading edge due to **swarming.**
- The toxigenicity is established by inoculating in mice and looking for signs of ascending tetanus.

**Treatment**

- **Wound debridement.**
- **Passive immunization** with antitetanus serum (ATS) which is a tetanus antitoxin.
- **Antibiotic therapy** in the form of Penicillin.
- **Supportive care.**

**Prevention**

Prevention involves **active immunization** in infancy with **tetanus toxoid** followed by booster doses.

**C. botulinum**

- These are gram-positive bacilli, are non-capsulated and **motile** by a peritrichate flagella.
- They possess oval subterminal spores.
- It grows well and produces β-haemolytic colonies on blood agar (except type G).

**Toxigenicity and Virulence**

- It produces a neurotoxin, **botulinum toxin** which is the most toxic substance known to man.
- On the basis of serological diversity among the toxins, they have been divided into 7 serological types (Type A-G).
- The toxins (A-F) acts by **inhibiting** the release of **acetylcholine** at the neuromuscular junction inhibiting neurotransmission at the cholinergic synapses. This leads to flaccid paralysis. Toxin G is not associated with any disease.

Pathogenesis and clinical disease

| *Infection caused* | *Pathogenesis* | *Clinical disease* |
|---|---|---|
| **Food-borne botulism** | Associated with processed and home prepared food especially meat and fish products.<br>It is due to ingestion of preformed toxin and the most common are toxin type A, B and E. | Symptoms begin after 18-36 hours of ingestion of food and include vomiting, dysphagia, diplopia, urinary retention, constipation.<br>Death occurs due to respiratory failure.<br>Paralysis is **descending** in character. |
| **Wound botulism** | Systemic intoxication caused by the toxin elaborated in the wound.<br>Most common types are A or B. | The symptoms are same as food-borne botulism except the GIT symptoms. |
| **Infant botulism** | Due to ingestion of spores by infants leading to the elaboration of the toxin in the intestines.<br>The common source is honey (fed to infants at birth).<br>Others are soil and household dust. | Affected infant presents with weakness and flaccid paralysis (**floppy child syndrome**). Symptoms are similar to food-borne botulism. |

## Laboratory Diagnosis

- The detection of the botulinum organism in faeces or sample of consumed food helps in diagnosis. *C. botulinum* can be isolated on egg yolk agar, blood agar and CMB. It is further identified on the basis of Gram staining, fluorescent antibody test and biochemical reactions.
- The best confirmatory test is the neutralization of the toxin detected in the patient's serum by antitoxin using toxin-antitoxin test in mice.

## Treatment

- **Supportive therapy-** to ensure ventilation, giving lavage and saline enemas.
- **Penicillin** is the antibiotic of choice.
- **Antitoxin-** use of polyvalent antitoxin against common types A,B and E can be given.

## Clostridium difficile

- They are gram-positive bacilli, are **motile** with peritrichate flagella and have subterminal or terminal spores.
- It is an obligate anaerobe and grows well on blood agar. The other media used for its isolation are cycloserine mannitol blood agar (CMBA) and cycloserine cefoxitin egg yolk fructose agar (CCFA).
- It liquefies gelatine and hydrolyses aesculin.

**Toxigenicity and pathogenesis**

*C. difficile* produces disease by the elaboration of two toxins:

- **Toxin A (enterotoxin)**—It induces an inflammatory reaction in rabbit intestine leading to fluid accumulation. It is primarily responsible for diarrhoea.
- **Toxin B (cytotoxin):** It is responsible for restructuring of the cell cytoskeleton.

**Clinical disease**

**Antibiotic-associated diarrhoea**: It is associated with imbalance of the normal intestinal flora due to administration of broad-spectrum antibiotics (e.g., clindamycin, cephalosporins, ampicillin).

The patient develops mild to severe watery diarrhoea (sometimes bloody) after 5-10 days of antibiotic therapy.

**Pseudomembranous colitis**: It can develop in severe cases as a consequence to the release of cytotoxin.

It can lead to life-threatening complications of fulminant pancolitis, megacolon and perforation.

The exudates consist of fibrin, mucin and polymorphonuclear leucocytes attached to the mucosal surface, which has a membrane like appearance.

## Diagnosis

- **Culture and isolation** of *C. difficile* from stool samples.
- **Demonstration of the cytotoxin.**
- **Latex agglutination** for *C. difficile* antigen in faecal supernate.

## Treatment

- Discontinuation of the prescribed antibiotic.
- The antibiotics of choice are **metronidazole and vancomycin.**

**Other Clostridium**

| *Organism* | *Morphology* | *Toxins produced* | *Associated disease* |
|---|---|---|---|
| ***C. septicum*** | Gram-positive, motile, subterminal spores. | α, β, γ and δ toxins and fibrinolysin. | Gas gangrene in man along with other clostridia. |
| ***C. histolyticum*** | Gram-positive, weakly motile, subterminal spores | α, β, γ, δ and ε toxins | Gas gangrene in man. |
| ***C. sordelli*** | Gram-positive, motile, terminal or subterminal spores | A lecithinase (similar to alpha toxin of *C perfringens)*, haemolysin and fibrinolysin. | Clostridial myonecrosis in man. |

Other organisms causing gas gangrene include: *C. sporogenes, C. haemolyticum* and *C. novyi.*

# BRANCHING GRAM-POSITIVE BACILLI

## ACTINOMYCETES (SEE TABLE 2.1)

Actinomycetes are gram-positive pleomorphic bacteria that often form branching filaments.

They comprise four potentially pathogenic genera: **Actinomyces, Nocardia, Streptomyces and Actinomadura.**

These organisms are closely related to mycobacteria and were earlier classified as fungi.

## NON-BRANCHING GRAM-POSITIVE BACILLI

| *Organism* | *Habitat* | *Mode of transmission* | *Disease caused* |
|---|---|---|---|
| **Erysipelothrix** | More common in animals, not found as normal flora in humans. | Abrasion or wound of skin with animal exposure | *Erysipeloid* localized skin infection with systemic manifestations. |
| **Arcanobacterium** | Normal flora of skin and pharynx. | Uncertain, probably by person's endogenous strains. | Pharyngitis, cellulitis and other skin infections (Reverse cAMP test positive). |
| **Gardenella** | Normal vagina flora in humans. | Endogenous strains. | Bacterial vaginosis. |
| **Lactobacillus** | Normal flora of mouth, GIT and female genital tract. | Endogenous strains. | Most frequently isolated as contaminant. Causes bacteraemia in immunocompromised |

# GRAM-NEGATIVE BACTERIA

## GRAM-NEGATIVE COCCI

## NEISSERIA

### General Characters

- They are gram-negative cocci, which are kidney-shaped and are often seen as diplococci.
- Most of them possess pili, are capsulated, non-motile and non-sporing.

**Table 2.1:** Differentiating characteristics of Actinomycetes

| *Characteristics* | *Actinomyces* | *Nocardia* | *Streptomyces* | *Actinomadura* |
|---|---|---|---|---|
| **Staining characters** | Gram-positive and acid-fast | Gram-positive and acid-fast (both weakly). | Gram-positive and non -acid-fast. | Gram-positive and non-acid fast. |
| **Cultural characters** | Strict or facultative anaerobes. Grow on brain heart infusion agar (BHIA), blood agar with 5-10 % $CO_2$ at 37° C in 10-14 days | Strict aerobes. It grows on nutrient agar, Sabourand Dextrose Agar (SDA) and BHIA at 37° C in 3 weeks. | Strict aerobes. Grows on SDA and BHIA. | Strict aerobes. Grows on SDA and BHIA to form leathery colonies. |
| **Epidemiology** | Part of normal flora (oropharynx and GIT). | Prevalent in soil Occasionally in sputum of normal individuals. | Occasionally in sputum and water. | Prevalent in soil. |
| **Pathogenic species** | *Actinomyces israelii* | *Nocardia brasiliensis* and *N. asteroides* | | *A. madurae* |

*Contd.*

*Contd.*

| | | | | |
|---|---|---|---|---|
| **Clinical disease** | Chronic suppurative infection-actinomycosis. 3 main sites of primary ifection-cervicofacial (mandible or maxilla), thoracic (lung) and abdominal (pelvic). | Opportunistic pulmonary disease, usually in immunocompromised. Dissemination via lymphohematogenous route can occur. | Causes mycetoma-sub cutaneous abscess of lower extremities with draining sinuses. | Causes chronic and destructive infection of skin & subcutaneous tissue, characterized by multiple sinuses and fistula (**madura foot**). |
| **Diagnosis** | **Microscopy**- pus discharge with granules-stained with Gram stain and ZN stain with 1% $H_2SO_4$ for decolourization. **Culture**-isolation on BHIA, blood agar. | **Microscopy**- stained with Gram stain and ZN stain with 1% $H_2SO_4$ for decolourization. **Culture**-isolation on BHIA, SDA, blood agar. | **Microscopy**-Gram stain of granules. **Culture**-on BHIA and SDA. | **Microscopy**-Gram stain of granules. **Culture**-on BHIA and SDA. |
| **Treatment** | High doses of Penicillin for 12-18 months. | Sulphonamides and amphotericin. | Sulphonamides and amphotericin | Sulphonamides and amphotericin |

- They are oxidase positive and aerobic. They have exacting growth requirements and grow in media enriched with serum or blood.
- Best growth is seen on chocolate agar (heated blood agar) in the presence of 5-10% $CO_2$ at 37° C.

## Classification

The genus *Neisseria* includes two pathogenic species- *N. meningitidis* and *N. gonorrhoeae*, as well as several non-pathogenic species.

The non-pathogenic species are found as normal commensals in the upper respiratory tract.

### *N. meningitidis*

- They are gram-negative cocci, that occur in pairs and most of the fresh isolates are **capsulated**. It is one of the most virulent human pathogens and an etiologic agent of meningitis.
- They can be isolated on blood agar and chocolate agar under 5-10 % $CO_2$ and increased humidity at 37° C.
- *N. meningitidis* is oxidase positive and **utilize glucose and maltose** with the production of acid but no gas.

## Classification

Meningococci can be grouped into 13 serogroups according to antigenic differences in capsular polysaccharides. The serogroups are A, B, C, D, X, Y, Z, 29e, W-135, H, I, K,L.

Most meningeal diseases are caused by serogroups **A, B, C** and to a small proportion by Y, W-135, X, Z and 29E.

## Virulence and Pathogenicity

**Adhesion factors:** The pili serve as adhesion factors for oropharyngeal mucosa and mediate attachment to meningeal tissue as well.

**Capsule:** The capsular polysaccharide contributes to invasiveness of meningococci by decreasing phagocytosis.

**Lipopolysaccharide (LPS, endotoxin):** It is similar to those of other gram-negative bacilli. The meningococci produce vesicles of LPS and liberate them extracellularly. This induces an inflammatory response and causes vascular necrosis. It can produce both localized and generalized **Shwartzman reaction.**

**IgA1 protease:** This cleaves IgA at hinge region and inactivates it.

**Outer membrane proteins:** There are classes of OMP, of which class 5 helps in attachment to host cells.

Clinical disease

| *Stage of disease* | *Pathogenesis* | *Clinical symptoms* |
|---|---|---|
| **First stage** | The organism is present in nasopharynx and causes infection. | Asymptomatic to minor self-limiting illness. |
| **Second stage** | Meningococci enter bloodstream via cervical lymph nodes. | Fever, malaise and petechial skin lesions.<br>It may also cause DIC and septic shock, other complications as gangrene of digits and necrosis, bilateral haemorrhage of adrenals-**Waterhouse Friederichsen syndrome.** |
| **Third stage** | It involves infection of the meninges. The route of infection is controversial-can be via bloodstream (most accepted), along perineural sheath or through cribriform plate. | Severe headache, fever, stiff neck, vomiting and neurological signs (delirium and confusion). |

## Epidemiology

*N. meningitidis* is found in nasopharynx in 5-10 % of healthy individuals.

During the epidemics, the carrier rate can group to 20-90%, more among household contacts.

The infection is highly contagious and disseminated by droplet infection, direct contact and rarely by fomites.

## Laboratory Diagnosis

**Direct examination:** The CSF is turbid, under pressure and with high polymorphonuclear count, **Microscopy**-on Gram staining

**Gram-negative diplococci** surrounded by a pink halo can be seen inside polymorphs and also extracellularly.

**Rapid detection**: **Ag detection** can be done with polyvalent antimeningococcal serum. The methods used include CIEP and latex agglutination.

**Culture**: The samples to be collected include CSF, blood, aspirate from skin lesion, throat and other swabs.

In delay in transport, **Stuart's medium** is used as transport medium.

The organism can be isolated on BA, Chocolate agar or trypticase soy broth (for blood culture).

**Thayer Martin** selective medium is used when isolating from a mixture of organisms.

## Treatment

**Penicillin** in high doses, given intravenously or intrathecally, is the treatment of choice.

Other antibiotic of choice in penicillin sensitive individuals include Ceftriaxone and Chloramphenicol.

## Prophylaxis

**Chemoprophylaxis** is done with Rifampicin and Ciprofloxacin in individuals coming in close contact with patients.

**Immunoprophylaxis:** A quadrivalent vaccine constituted by capsular polysaccharide of serotype A, C, Y and W-135 is available.

No vaccine is available against group B as it is a poor immunogen.

Conjugate vaccine with A and C polysaccharide with diphtheria toxin is under evaluation.

### *Neisseria gonorrhoeae*

- It is similar to *Neisseria meningitidis* in morphology and staining characters.
- They are more difficult to grow than meningococci, can be isolated on chocolate agar.
- **Thayer Martin medium and modified Thayer Martin media** are important selective media for their isolation.
- Gonococci are oxidase positive and **utilize glucose** with the production of acid only.

### Classification

They are divided into serotypes based upon outer membrane proteins. **Auxotyping** is done on the basis of amino acid requirement and there are more than 30 auxotypes.

### Antigenic Structure and Virulence

**Pili-** gonococci are involved in adherence of bacteria to host cell. They are also antiphagocytic.

**Outer membrane proteins (OMPs) :** They have OMP named proteins I, II and III.

- Protein I is the basis of **serotyping** of gonococci.
- Protein II, also known as **opacity associated protein**, helps in adherence of the bacteria to host cells.
- Protein III along with protein I help in formation of porins.

**Endotoxins:** It plays a role in disseminated infection, is less toxic than that of *N. meningitidis.*

**Peptidoglycan:** It has inflammatory properties.

**IgA1 protease:** It helps evade mucosal immunity.

## Pathogenesis and Clinical Disease

It enters the body through mucous membrane of genitourinary tract by penetrating the columnar epithelium.

**Local infections**

| | |
|---|---|
| **Males** | |
| **Urethritis** | Predominant infection.<br>S/S: urethral discharge and dysuria. |
| Complications | Epididymitis, prostatitis, disseminated infection, stricture formation and fibrosis. |
| **Females** | |
| **Cervicitis** | Predominant infection.<br>S/S: dyspareunia, dysuria, chronic pain, sterility and ectopic pain. |
| Complications | PID, urethritis, infection of Fallopian tubes, ovaries and Bartholin's glands. |
| **Anorectal infections** | Seen in both sexes (common in homosexuals). Occur due to autoinoculation. |
| **Ophthalmia neonatorum** | Conjunctivitis in newborns acquired during passage through infected birth canal. |
| **Pharyngeal gonorrhoea** | Due to orogenital contact. |
| **Disseminated infection** | Due to haematogenous spread. |

## Epidemiology

Person to person spread occurs via sexual intercourse.

Infection can spread from mother to child during childbirth.

Rarely, infection spreads from inanimate objects.

## Laboratory Diagnosis

In women, **endocervical swab** is the most suitable sample.

In males, **urethral discharge** is the most suitable sample.

### Direct detection

**Microscopy** on Gram staining **intracellular gram-negative diplococci** in symptomatic individuals is usually diagnostic. Positive samples are more common in symptomatic men (90%) than in women (50-60%) due to confusion caused by their normal flora.

**Direct immunofluorescence (for Ag detection)**-using fluorescent antibodies tagged *N. gonorrhoeae* and by using DNA and RNA probes (for nucleic acid detection) are other rapid methods.

**Culture for isolation**

It is cultured on **Thayer Martin** or **modified Thayer Martin** media in the presence of 5-10% $CO_2$ at temperature of 35-36° C.

Oxidase positive gram-negative diplococci can be confirmed by biochemical reactions.

**Serology:** It is useful for chronic and disseminated infections. Detection of IgM, IgG and IgA antibodies can be done by ELISA, RIA and haemagglutination tests.

## Treatment

Though Penicillin was the treatment of choice earlier, resistance has been demonstrated in the form of **chromosomally mediated resistant *N. gonorrhoeae* (CMRNG).** These strains show a higher MIC. In such cases, larger doses of penicillin preceded by probenecid is recommended.

**Penicillinase producing *N gonorrhoeae*** (**PPNG**) were isolated in 1976 from US and England. The resistance is due to β-lactamase production. Penicillin is ineffective in these patients and alternate drugs in the form of tetracycline and cephalosporins are administered.

Ophthalmia neonatorum- 1% tetracycline or .5% erythromycin is applied.

## MORAXELLA

These are gram-negative, oxidase positive aerobic diplococci. The pathogenic species is *Moraxella catarrhalis* which causes **otitis media** in humans. Previously known as *Branhamella catarrhalis.*

# GRAM-NEGATIVE BACILLI

## HAEMOPHILUS

- The genus *Haemophilus* ('hemal' meaning blood and 'philos' means friendly) includes several human pathogens of which *H. influenzae* is the most important.
- These organisms are non-motile, non-sporing, gram-negative coccobacilli which are pleomorphic.
- They require one or both of 2 accessory growth factors (X and V) present in blood. Other species of medical importance include: *H. ducreyi, H. parainfluenzae, H. aegytius, H. aphrophilus and H. parphrophilus.*

### H. influenzae

They are gram-positive coccobacilli which are non-motile and difficult to stain.

Staining with carbol fuschin for 10-15 minutes gives better results.

A few virulent stains possess capsule.

**Growth characters**

*H. influenzae* is a fastidious organism that grows better in 5-10% $CO_2$ at temperature between 35-37°C.

Accessory growth factors are essential for its growth. These include:

**X factor:** It is a heat stable protoporphyrin that is required for the synthesis of iron containing respiratory enzymes as cytochrome c, cytochrome oxidase, peroxidase and catalase.

**V factor:** It is an NADP, which is essential for oxidation-reduction process in the bacterial cells.

These factors are found within the RBCs. Hence regular blood agar that contains intact RBCs (and also NADase) does not support its growth as the factor V is inadequate.

The media best suited for its isolation are:

**Chocolate agar:** It is formed by heating blood agar at 80-90° C which leads to lysis of erythrocytes and release of X and V factors. Heating also leads to inactivation of NADase.

**Blood agar:** *H. influenzae* grows well on blood agar if *Staphylococcus aureus* is simultaneously streaked on it. The colonies are large and well developed along the streak of *S. aureus* and are smaller farther away. This phenomenon is known as **satellitism**. The lysis of RBCs surrounding the *S. aureus* streak provide X factor while V factor is secreted by *S. aureus.*

**Other media** used include **Levinthal agar** and **Filde's blood digest agar,** both of which are transparent media containing digested blood.

*H. influenzae* is catalase and oxidase positive, and on the basis of production of indole, urease and ornithine decarboxylase activity are divided into 6 biotypes.

## Classification

Some strains produce a polysaccharide capsule, which is the basis of capsular typing and division into **6 serotypes (a-f).** Most of the infections are caused by serotype b.

## Virulence and Pathogenicity

**Pili:** They assist the organism in attachment to the epithelial cells.

**Capsular polysaccharide:** The capsular polysaccharide of *Haemophilus influenzae* type b is constituted by phosphoribosylribitol phosphate (PRP). The capsule has antiphagocytic properties.

**Membranous lipooligosaccharides:** It is similar but shorter than LPS of *E. coli.* It helps in attachment and invasiveness.

**Outer membrane proteins:** They also help in attachment.

**IgA proteases:** They inactivate the secondary antibodies.

## Epidemiology

The non-capsulated strains of *Haemophilus influenzae* are found in healthy adults in the nasopharynx and oropharynx (25-80%). *Haemophilus* type b constitutes 5-10% while 1-2% is type c-f.

The usual portal of entry is the upper respiratory tract.

## Clinical Disease

Infections caused by *Haemophilus influenzae*

| | *Infections* | *Age group affected* |
|---|---|---|
| **Invasive infections** | Meningitis | Children between 6 months to 2 years. |
| | Otitis media and sinusitis | Young children. |
| | Acute bacterial epiglottitis | 2-5 years. |
| | Cellulitis (face and neck). | < 2 years. |
| | Bacteremia (mainly HI ) type b | Children. |
| | Pneumonia | Infants. |
| | Septic arthritis. | < 2 years. |
| **Non-invasive infections** Usually associated with underlying and/or physical abnormality. Mainly due to non-capsular strains. | Otitis media, sinusitis, chronic bronchitis, bronchiectasis and conjunctivitis. | Usually in children. |

## Laboratory Diagnosis

**Direct examination:** Gram stain of CSF and other specimen show poorly stained gram-negative coccobacilli.

Immunofluorescence and Quellung reaction can be done for capsular detection.

Latex agglutination and coagglutination for type b capsular antigen detection can also be performed.

**Culture:** CSF or other samples are plated on blood agar with staphylococcal streak or chocolate agar with 5-10% $CO_2$ and incubated overnight at 37° C.

## Treatment

A wide range of antibiotics can be used for the treatment. Tetracycline, Ampicillin with Chloramphenicol and third generation cephalosporins are used. In β-lactamase producing type b strains, chloramphenicol or third generation cephalosporins are used.

**Rifampicin** is used for chemoprophylaxis.

**Purified type b PRP vaccine** induces good antibody response in children older than 18 months. Conjugate vaccines with diphtheria and tetanus toxoid are also under trial.

Other important Haemophilus species

| *Organism* | *Growth requirement* | *Virulence factors* | *Spectrum of disease* |
|---|---|---|---|
| *H. ducreyi* | Requires X factor only. Grows only on special media. | Uncertain, but capsular factors, pili and certain toxins help in attachment and penetration. | STD. Chancroid, generalized lesions that progress from tender papules to **painful ulcers.** Inguinal lymphadenitis is common. |
| *H. aegyptius* | Requires X and V factor, grows on Chocolate agar. | Uncertain, probably similar to HI. | Purulent conjunctivitis, Brazilian purpuric fever that has increased mortality in children between 1 to 4 years. It is characterized by symptoms similar to meningococcaemia. |
| *H. parainfluenzae* | Requires only V factor. Grows on chocolate agar. | Has a low pathogenicity. | Can cause pharyngitis, endocarditis and bronchopulmonary infection in patients with cystic fibrosis. |

*Contd.*

*Contd.*

| | | |
|---|---|---|
| *H. aphrophilus* | Requires X factor, grows on chocolate agar. | Jaw infection and endocarditis. |
| *H. paraphrophilus* | Requires only V factor. | Commensal and usually non-pathogenic. |
| *H haemolyticus* | Requires both X and V factor. | Commensal and usually non-pathogenic. |

## BORDETELLA

It consists of gram-positive coccobacilli that are strict aerobes, are non-sporing and most of the strains are haemolytic.

There are 6 species of which, ***Bordetella pertussis,*** the causative agent of whooping cough is the most pathogenic. The other species are:

- ***B. parapertussis:*** causes mild cases of whooping cough.
- ***B. bronchoseptica*:** causes bronchopneumonia in animals and occasionally infection resembling whooping cough in man.
- ***B. avium:*** found in birds, causes rhinotracheitis in them.
- ***B. pertussis*** and ***B. parapertussis*** are non-motile, while the others are motile.

### Bordetella pertussis

#### General characters

- It is an obligate aerobe, non-motile and is sensitive to unsaturated fatty acids, sulfides and peroxidases.
- It is weakly oxidase positive.
- It is usually isolated on **Bordet-Gengou media,** which contains potato starch, 50% blood and glycerol. Starch acts by neutralizing the effect of toxic materials; while glycerol is the stabilizing agent.

- The media should be immediately involuted with the sample, but in case of a delay **Amie's charcoal** media (charcoal neutralizes the inhibitory materials) can be used.
- The growth takes 3-5 days to appear. The colonies are haemolytic; resemble **bisected pearls or mercury drops**.

### Virulence

**Adhesion:** Adherence of *B. pertussis* to ciliated epithelial cells of the upper respiratory tract is mediated by filamentous haemagglutinins.

Toxins

| *Toxins* | *Action* |
|---|---|
| **Pertussis toxin** | Major toxin produced by *Bordetella pertussis.*<br>Acts by activation of adenyl cyclase, leading to increased cAMP that causes cell dysfunction.<br>Leads to leucocytosis, increased histamine and serotonin production and increased insulin synthesis. |
| **Adenylate cyclase like toxin** | Leads to intracellular increase in cAMP to support the intracellular survival of the bacteria.<br>Inhibits chemotaxis and superoxide burst in polymorph leucocytes. |
| **LPS endotoxin** | It is similar to gram-negative bacterial endotoxins, leading to pyrogenicity and Schwartzman reactivity. |
| **Tracheal cytotoxin** | It destroys the tracheal epithelium leading to the characteristic cough. |
| **Others** | |
| **HLT** | It causes increase in inflammatory reaction. |
| **Haemolysin** | It is responsible for haemolysis on Bordet-Gengou media. |

## Pathogenesis and Clinical Disease

*Bordetella pertussis* is an obligate human parasite of the upper respiratory tract. The symptoms of whooping cough are related to the destruction of the ciliated epithelial cells of bronchi and trachea whereas the systemic symptoms are caused by the pertussis toxin.

Spectrum of diseases

| *Stages* | *Pathogenesis* | *Clinical spectrum* |
|---|---|---|
| **Prodromal or Catarrhal stage Incubation Period** 7-14 days | Contagious stage with increase in organisms in the upper respiratory tract. | Low grade fever, rhinorrhoea and irritating cough. |
| **Paroxysmal stage** After 1-2 weeks | Lasts for 6-8 weeks. Patient is non-infectious after 6 weeks. | Paroxysmal coughing episodes-spasmodic phase of cough followed by rapid inrush **(whoop)** or air. |
| **Convale-scence complications** | Lasts for 1-3 weeks. Non-infectious. | Decrease in frequency of cough. |
| **Pulmonary** | | Bronchitis, pneumonia as secondary infection. |
| **Neurological** | | Encephalopathy or convulsions following infections. |

## Laboratory Diagnosis

*Bordetella pertussis* can be adequately collected from nasopharynx during the catarrhal phase by a **pernasal swab** impregnated with calcium alginate.

Cotton swabs are not used as cotton is inhibitory to bacteria.

The sample is inoculated onto Bordet-Gengou media and growth is confirmed by morphological, microscopic and biochemical tests.

**Rapid diagnosis:** Direct immunofluorescence for Antigen detection in nasopharyngeal swabs can be done.

**Bordetella Antibodies in serum:** Can be done by ELISA, Latex agglutination and indirect haemagglutination.

## Treatment

The drug of choice is **Erythromycin** which is coupled with supportive measures.

## Prevention

**DPT vaccine**, which contains killed pertussis vaccine, is protective. It is given at 6, 10 and 14 weeks followed by a booster at one and a half year of age. Complications, mainly neurological, are rare.

**Acellular subunit vaccine** is able to overcome the neurological complications is currently under trial. This contains inactivated pertussis toxin (PT), filamentous haemagglutinins (FHA) and agglutinogens 1, 2, 3.

## BRUCELLA

- These are gram-negative coccobacilli, which are **non-motile,** intracellular and require blood or serum enriched complex media (as serum dextrose agar) for growth. It grows at 37°C in 48 hours.
- They are **strict aerobes**, capnophilic (require 5-10% $CO_2$). It is catalase and urease positive while some species are also oxidase positive.
- These are essentially animal pathogens that are sporadically transmitted to and cause infections in humans—**zoonotic bacteria**.

### Classification

The main species that can cause human infections are ***B. melitensis*** (the classical species of the genus), ***B. abortus, B. suis*** *and* ***B. canis.***

These are essentially animal pathogens that are sporadically transmitted to and cause infections in humans- **zoonotic bacteria**.

### Classification

The main species that can cause human infections are ***B. melitensis*** (the classical species of the genus), ***B. abortus, B. suis*** *and* ***B. canis.***

| | |
|---|---|
| *B. melitensis* | It is pathogenic for sheep and goats. Man is also susceptible. |
| *B. abortus* | Causes abortion in cattle. Brucellosis in man. |
| *B. suis* | Natural parasite of pig. Man can get infected too. |
| *B. canis* | Abortions in dogs. Occasional pyrexial illness in man. |

They are divided into various species and biotypes on the basis of $CO_2$ requirement, $H_2S$ production, urease production, growth in the presence of dyes and agglutination by monospecific antiserum.

## Epidemiology

*B. melitensis* is the most pathogenic species for man. Infection in animals occurs through the GIT, skin and mucous membrane of conjunctiva.

## Infection in Humans

- Direct contact with animal or animal tissue in farmers, dairy workers, abbaittoir workers and veterinarians.
- Ingestion of contaminated food (meat or infected milk).
- Inhalation of aerosolized organisms.
- Accidental ingestion/inhalation in laboratory.

## Virulence

It is based upon:

- Ability to resist phagocytosis.
- Ability to survive and multiply intracellularly by evading the host immune response.
- The bacteria localize in reticuloendothelial system, eliciting a granulomatous host response.

## Clinical Disease

The incubation period of the disease is 3-16 days.

### Acute brucellosis

It is characterized by fever, headache, constipation with myalgia and arthralgia. The fever and other symptoms show periodic nocturnal pattern over weeks of exacerbation and relapses, hence the name **undulant fever.**

### Chronic brucellosis

If the disease persists for greater than 6 months, it is referred to as chronic brucellosis.

## Laboratory Diagnosis

Culture and isolation are necessary to confirm diagnosis.

**Blood culture is the most definitive method-** the chances of collection of brucella during the rising phase in pyrexia are high.

The organism can also be isolated from bone marrow aspirate and liver biopsy.

Blood culture is done on **Serum Dextrose Broth (SDB)** at 37°C in the presence of 5-10% $CO_2$. Since the growth takes 8 weeks to appear, **a 2-phase system or Casteneda method** of blood culture is used. In this, both liquid and solid media are used within the same bottle and subculture is done every 3-5 days by tilting the bottle. This prevents chances of contamination and decreases risk of infection to the laboratory personnel.

## Serology

IgM antibodies are the first to appear (7-10 days) followed by IgG and IgA. The detection of these is supportive in diagnosis.

- Agglutination for IgM- for acute brucellosis.
- ELISA and complement fixation test for both IgM and IgG- for chronic brucellosis.

**Other tests:**

**Standard tube agglutination (SAT) test:** A single titre =160 by SAT serves as a presumptive evidence.

RIA, ELISA and Coomb's test.

**Brucellin skin test:** To detect delayed type IV hypersensitivity- gives a past history of exposure.

**Infection in animals**

- **Rose Bengal card test.**
- **Rapid plate agglutination test.**
- **Milk ring test:** Antibody detection in pooled milk samples.

## Treatment

**Tetracycline** with **streptomycin** is the drug of choice.

## Control and Prevention

Herd vaccination (live attenuated *B. abortus* strain 19 vaccine).

Pasteurization of animal milk.

Wearing of protective clothing by persons handling animals.

# CAMPYLOBACTER

## General Characters

These are gram-negative, curved rods arranged in pairs which are **comma** or S-shaped (or **gull wing** shaped). They are **microaerophilic** (grow best in 5% $O_2$), **capnophilic** (require 10% $CO_2$ for growth) and **thermophilic** (grow best at 42°C).

They are non-sporing, oxidase positive and motile by means of single polar unsheathed flagella.

They cause two major groups of disease—fetal inflammation of cattle and sheep, and **acute enterocolitis of humans.**

## Classification

**Campylobacter** consists of 15 species, but the most important are *C. jejuni, C. coli* and *C. fetus.*

Pathogenesis and virulence factors

| *Factors* | *Role in virulence* |
|---|---|
| Lipopolysaccharides | Endotoxic activity |
| Cytopathic extracellular toxins | Their significance in human disease is not defined. |
| Cholera-like enterotoxins | |
| Motility and flagella | Determinants of attachment and invasion. |

## Epidemiology

**Campylobacter** are zoonotic bacteria with many animal reservoirs. Humans are infected via food or water contaminated with animal faeces.

Human to human transmission occurs by **fecal-oral route.**

## Clinical Disease

- Enterocolitis is primarily caused by *C. jejuni* and manifest as acute onset of crampy abdominal pain, profuse diarrhoea followed by bloody stools and accompanied with headache, malaise and fever.
- **Campylobacter** is also associated with **Guillian-Barre syndrome**, an acute inflammatory demyelinating polyneuropathy associated with axonal motor neuropathy.
- It is also associated with autoimmune diseases as **reactive arthritis** and **Reiter's syndrome.**

## Laboratory Diagnosis

- **Direct examination:** Gram stained smears of faecal material show comma-shaped gram-negative bacteria.
- **Culture:** The sample should be immediately transported to the laboratory and in case of a delay Cary-Blair's transport media is used.
- For optimal recovery, **Campylobacter** requires, microaerophilic atmosphere containing 5% $O_2$, 10% $CO_2$ and 85% $N_2$. The culture is done on selective media and the plates are incubated at 42°C.
- Several selective media are in use, as **Skirrow's medium** containing vancomycin, polymixin B and trimethoprim to inhibit other bacteria. Other media containing antimicrobials and other inhibitory compounds are also used as selective media.

## Treatment

Erythromycin and ciprofloxacin are effective against *C. jejuni* enterocolitis.

# HELICOBACTER

## General Characters

- These are gram-negative spiral-shaped (helical) rods, which are capnophilic, microaerophilic and strongly urease positive.
- They are motile by means of single or multiple unipolar/bipolar sheathed flagella.
- *H. pylori* are associated with antral gastritis, duodenal or gastric ulcers and gastric carcinomas.

## Pathogenesis and Virulence

*H. pylori* overlie gastric type and not intestinal type of epithelium. It is found deep in the mucous layer overlying the epithelium.

| *Factors* | *Role in virulence* |
|---|---|
| Urease (production of ammonia) | Cause damage to the mucosa and predispose to gastritis and peptic ulcer. |
| Protease | |
| Inflammatory response | |
| Motility | Spread of infection. |
| Cytotoxin | Cause vacuolation in cultured gastric cells, which predisposes to gastric ulcer or gastric carcinoma |

## Clinical Disease

*H. pylori* infection is associated with chronic gastritis, peptic ulcer and gastric carcinoma that present with recurrent pain in upper abdomen and bleeding in the upper git. This can be associated with nausea, vomiting, pain, fever and other non-specific symptoms.

## Diagnosis

**Direct examination:** The organism can be seen on Gram stained smears of biopsy specimen of the gastric mucosa.

Other methods of detection include immunofluorescent acridine orange, histochemical, Giemsa or special silver stains.

Molecular methods as PCR can be used for antigen detection.

Detection of *H. pylori* antigen in stool samples is done to evaluate the prognosis of patients treated.

**Tests of urease activity:** These are special tests that aid in diagnosis of infection.

***In vitro* testing of biopsy tissue:** This is done by testing biopsy tissue for urease activity by placing it on to urea containing medium with colour indicators. If *H. pylori* are present, urease splits urea liberating ammonia resulting in pH shift that causes a color change. This test is also known as **Campylobacter like organism (CLO) test.**

**Urea breath test:** A non-invasive method is, detecting radiolabelled $CO_2$ after oral administration of [$^{13}C$] urea (due to activity of enzyme urease) in the breath of the person.

**Urine test:** Breakdown of $^{15}N$ labelled urea yields $CO_2$ and $^{15}N$ labelled ammonia that can be traced by mass spectrometry.

**Culture:** Same as **Campylobacter**.

## Treatment

- A combination of antacids and one or two broad-spectrum antibiotics are the treatment of choice.
- Omeprezole, a proton pump inhibitor, is the preferred antacid.
- Antibiotics used include metronidazole, tetracycline, amoxicillin or clarithromycin with bismuth subsalisylate for 1-3 weeks are used.

# PASTEURELLA

## General Characters

These are gram-negative coccobacilli, which are non-motile, capsulated at 37°C and show **bipolar staining** in tissues with methylene blue.

It grows well on nutrient agar and forms non-haemolytic colonies on blood agar.

### Classification

The pathogenic species is *P. multocida.*

It has 15 serotypes based upon the capsular antigenic typing.

### Pathogenesis and Clinical Disease

It is found in the respiratory tract of domestic animals and birds.

In humans, especially farmers are susceptible following bite by cats or dogs.

The infections caused include to cellulites, adenitis and osteomyelitis.

### Diagnosis

It is based on culture and biochemical testing.

### Treatment

It is sensitive to penicillin, tetracycline, erythromycin and streptomycin.

## FRANCISELLA

### General Characters

- These are small gram-negative pleomorphic coccobacilli, which are capsulated (virulence factor), non-motile and non-sporing
- They are strict aerobes and do not grow on ordinary media. It grows well on blood agar with glucose and cystine chloride, giving **droplet like colonies.**

### Pathogenesis and Clinical Disease

- The pathogenic species is *F. tularensis.* It is the etiological agent of tularaemia (acute zoonotic plague like disease of rodents and small mammals as rabbits).
- It is a **tick borne infection**.
- Man is the accidental host- transmission is air-borne or water-borne or through laboratories.

### Clinical Disease

The disease presents with influenza like or typhoidal symptoms. It is often accompanied with lymph-adenopathy, fever and malaise.

### Diagnosis

It is based on culture and antibody detection in sera of patients by slide or tube agglutination.

### Treatment

The drugs of choice are streptomycin and gentamicin.

## LEGIONELLACEAE

In the year 1976, following an American Legion convention in Philadelphia, many participants developed pneumonia. This disease was referred to as **Legionnaire's disease** and the causative agent as *Legionella pneumophila.*

### Morphology

*L. pneumophila* is Gram negative, pleomorphic, non-sporing, motile with one or more polar or subpolar flagella. It is difficult to stain with conventional bacteriological stains, but best stained in tissues by silver impregnation stains.

### Classification

Legionella contain many species, of which *L. pneumophila* is the most important. On the basis of direct or indirect immunofluorescence with slide agglutination, they can be divided into 15 serogroups. Most of the infections are due to serogroup 1.

### Pathogenicity and Virulence

It is an intracellular organism, and its major virulence is characterized by its ability to survive and multiply inside phagocytic cells.

## Toxins

An endotoxin and haemolysin, a cytotoxin and protease appear to be an important determinant of virulence.

## Clinical Disease

The infection has an incubation period of 2-10 days.

Infection may occur in two forms:

1. **Legionnaire's disease:** It is a patchy and diffuse or lobar pneumonia that can show extrapulmonary spread (kidney, liver, spleen). The clinical signs are non-specific as of fever, chills, headache and cough.
2. **Pontiac fever:** It is a self-limiting, flu-like syndrome without lung involvement.

## Epidemiology

*L. pneumophila* has a natural habitat in water. The organism can be isolated from **air-conditioning cooling** towers, cooling water systems, hot water systems.

Contaminated water can be a source of infection for persons inhaling mist from such sources.

## Laboratory Diagnosis

**Microscopy:** Rapid diagnosis can be made by **direct immunofluorescence** for antigen detection or silver staining of biopsy tissues or sputum.

Gram staining shows poor staining gram-negative rods in a normally sterile site.

**Culture and isolation:** The specimen is inoculated on buffered charcoal yeast extract agar **(BCYE agar)** and incubated at 36° C for up to 10 days.

Under microscope, the colonies have **cut glass appearance.**

**Serology:** Antibodies to *L. pneumophila* develop 6-8 days after clinical onset of infection and are detected by indirect fluorescent antibody test. A four fold rise in titre or ≥ 256 units is diagnostic.

## Treatment

It is sensitive to **Erythromycin** and **Rifampicin**. Penicillins and Cephalosporins are not effective since they produce β-lactamases.

**Doxycycline** is administered to patients who cannot tolerate erythromycin.

## PSEUDOMONADS

The name 'pseudomonads' is applied to gram-negative, aerobic non-sporulated rod-shaped bacteria that are motile (except ***Burkhoderia mallei***) by means of polar flagella. They are catalase and oxidase positive (except ***Stenotrophomonas maltophila)***. They are usually opportunistic pathogens and have an intrinsic capacity for tolerance to many deleterious agents, including antibiotics.

## Classification

The aerobic pseudomonads, on the basis of ribosomal RNA homology, are divided into 5 groups. These are:

| *Groups* | *Genus* | *Important species* |
|---|---|---|
| rRNA Group I | Pseudomonas | Fluorescent- *P. aeruginosa, P. putida, P. fluorescens, P. flavescens.*<br>Non-pigmented-*P. alcaligenes, P. stutzeri.* |
| rRNA Group II | Burkholderia and *B. cepacia.* | *B. mallei, B. pseudomallei* |
| rRNA Group III | Commamonas | |
| rRNA Group IV | Brevundimonas | |
| rRNA Group V | Stenotropho-monas, Xanthomonas | *S. maltophila.* |
| Not assigned | Sphingomonas | |

**Pigments:** Fluorescent pigments are characteristic of the fluorescent pseudomonads. A medium used to stimulate the pigment production is the **King B** medium.

| *Pigment* | *Nature* | *Organism producing it* |
|---|---|---|
| **Pyocyanin** | A blue, phenazine derivative, diffuses into the surrounding medium. It is water soluble **(Enhanced in King A media).** | Only *P. aeruginosa* (its production is diagnostic). |
| **Pyorubin** | Bright red, water soluble. | *P. aeruginosa* |
| **Pyomelanin** | Brown to black | *P. aeruginosa* |
| **Pyoverdin (fluorescein)** | Water soluble, yellowish. | Some strains of *P aeruginosa.* |
| **Carotenoid pigments** | Yellow or orange, . insoluble | Brevundimonas, Sphingomonas. |

## Pseudomonas aeruginosa

- Gram-negative strict aerobic bacilli that are non-sporing, non-capsulated and motile by polar flagella.
- It grows well in ordinary media. It produces smooth, translucent colonies on nutrient agar with a characteristic **fruity odour.**
- Many strains produce a **blue-green pigment.**
- It is resistant to quaternary ammonium compounds (e.g. cetrimide). **Cetrimide agar** with nalidixic acid and Irgasan containing media are used as selective media.

Antigenic structure and virulence

| | |
|---|---|
| **Extracellular enzymes and haemolysins** | |
| Proteases | They cause destructive vascular lesions, tissue necrosis and by destroying collagen help in the spread of infection. |
| Haemolysins | They destroy tissue surfactants and cause pulmonary atelectasis. |
| Phospholipase C and heat stable rhamnolipid | Degrade fats and inhibit monocyte chemotaxis. |
| Lipase | |
| **Extracellular toxins** | |
| Exotoxin A | Its action is similar to that of diphtheria toxin, acts by inhibiting protein synthesis by inactivating EF-2. |
| Exotoxin S | It is distinct from Exotoxin A and also inhibits phagocytic activity. |

*Contd.*

*Contd.*

| | |
|---|---|
| **Endotoxins** | It is an LPS with biological properties of enterobacterial LPS including pyrogenic action, Shwartzman reaction and lethality for mice. |
| **Pyocyanin** | It inhibits the mitochondrial enzymes in mammalian tissues, causes disruption of ciliated nasal epithelium and hence favours colonization of organisms in the nasal mucosa. |
| **Alginate capsule** | Produced by bacteria infecting the lungs-promote biofilm formation that confers protection from external environment as antibiotics and complement. |
| **Pilin and non-pilus adhesions** | Essential for initial colonisation of epithelial tissues. |

## Pathogenesis and Clinical Disease

They are mostly involved in opportunistic and nosocomial infections in individuals with predisposing conditions (e.g. extensive **burns**, trauma to skin or conjunctiva, urinary tract manipulations, **cystic fibrosis** etc).

The various infections with the predisposing conditions are:

| *Infection* | *Predisposing condition* |
|---|---|
| UTI | During catheterization and manipulations. |
| Acute purulent meningitis | During LP and after cranial infections. |
| Necrotizing pneumonia | Multiply on respiratory ventilators or enter lungs of dependent patients. |
| Septicaemia | Patients with leukaemia or on immunosuppressive therapy, newborns and old debilitated. |
| Endocarditis | Drug addicts. |
| Wound and burn infections | Extensive burn and trauma patients. |
| Chronic otitis media and otitis externa | Healthy children. |

### Cystic Fibrosis and Pseudomonas

Pseudomonas has an advanced ability to colonize patients with cystic fibrosis. A variety of factors contribute as: increase sialic acid content of saliva, increased mucin glycopeptides in patients with cystic fibrosis increase adhesion of pseudomonads, proteases damage to epithelial cells, increased release of exotoxin A, production of alginate capsule—all promote increased binding affinity for Pseudomonas and resistance to phagocytosis.

### Laboratory Diagnosis

- It requires culture and isolation.
- The specimen is collected from the site of infection and inoculated on to Mac Conkey agar and blood agar. The isolates are identified on the basis of colony morphology and biochemical characters.
- Serotyping (on the basis of O antigen typing) and pyocin (bacteriocin) typing can be carried out for further characterization.

### Treatment

*P. aeruginosa* are intrinsically resistant to most commonly employed antimicrobial agents. Many strains are sensitive to Carbenicillin, Azlocillin, Cefotaxime, Ceftazidine Tobramycin and Gentamicin.

### *Burkholderia pseudomallei*

- It consists of gram-negative, **bipolar staining bacilli** that are motile. It causes **meliodosis** (glanders like disease) in rats, guinea pigs and rabbits.
- Humans acquire infection by inhalation, inoculation and ingestion of foodstuff contaminated with infected animal excreta or bite of haematophagus animals.
- They survive in the reticuloendothelial system of humans.

- The infection presents as subclinical infection or benign pulmonary infection that resembles tuberculosis. Septicaemia and multiple organ abscesses may be seen.
- It is known as the **'Great Mimic'** as its imitates plague.
- In India, meliodosis has been reported from Maharashtra, Kerala, Tamil Nadu, Orissa and West Bengal.

## Laboratory Diagnosis

- Isolation from sputum, urine, pus or blood.
- IgG and IgM antibodies in patient's serum can be detected by ELISA and indirect haemagglutination.

## B. mallei

It was isolated from a horse dying of Glanders. It is small gram-negative, non-motile, aerobe and facultative anaerobe that can grow on ordinary culture media. It causes two types of lesions in horses, mules:

1. **Glanders:** The animal develops profuse catarrhal discharge from the nose, followed by nodule formation that can ulcerate.
2. **Farcy:** This is characterized by involvement of superficial lymph vessels and lymph nodes. The lymphatic vessels are thickened and stand out as cords.

Humans can be infected by contact of abraded skin with the discharge of infected animals. It may cause acute fulminant illness or abscess in respiratory tract or skin.

## B. cepacia

It is a gram-negative, motile, aerobic bacillus that accumulates poly-hydroxybutyrate as **granules** and produces reddish-purplish phenazine pigment.

It is a low grade pathogen and causes hospital associated infections. Its isolation from the lungs of debilitated patients is often **associated with cystic fibrosis.**

### Stenotrophomonas Maltophila

- It is a gram-negative, motile bacillus, which is **oxidase negative**.
- It is ubiquitous in nature and is associated with outbreak of infections in hospitals, particularly in ICUs. It is often recovered from bypass equipment, water baths and mechanical ventilators.
- These organisms are generally resistant to broad-spectrum antibiotics.
- Tetracycline, Doxycycline and third generation Cephalosporins have the highest activity against them.

## VIBRIONACEAE

The family Vibrionaceae includes three genera- Vibrio, Aeromonas and Plesiomonas.

The pre-eminent pathogen of this family is *Vibrio cholerae*.

### Vibrio

These are gram-negative **comma-shaped** bacilli, motile with single polar flagellum and are oxidase positive.

There are 36 nomenclature species in the genus *Vibrio.* The other pathogens are *Vibrio vulnificus and V. parahaemolyticus.*

### Classification

Classification is based on the antigenic characteristic of *Vibrio* species. It is defined by two features—the LPS ('O' or somatic antigen) and the flagellum (H or flagellar antigen). Currently, there are 24 serogroups of *V. cholerae.*

These can be identified as:

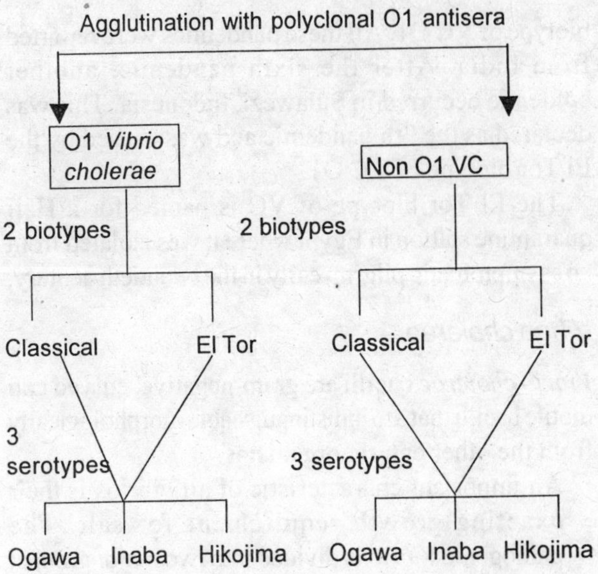


Ogawa is the most common serotype in India, Inaba being rare. Hikojima has never been isolated in India. In 1992, a new strain of *Vibrio cholerae* called the **O139 (Bengal strain)** appeared in the Indian sub-continent and SE Asia and caused a major epidemic.

## Epidemiology

Cholera is transmitted by faeco-oral contamination. Seasonal flooding, overcrowding and poor sanitation facilitates contamination of water supplies and outbreak of cholera.

Till recent past, VC O1 strains were the only ones associated with epidemic and pandemic cholera. Non O1 group is associated with isolated cases of cholera and small outbreaks of diarrhoea. The emergence of O139 as a major cause of epidemic cholera broke the cardinal rule of association of epidemic cholera with the O1 serogroup. Its appearance may represent the beginning of a new pandemic.

Between the years 1817 and 1920, 6 major pandemics occurred and were caused by the classical biotype of VC O1. All these pandemics were reported from India. After the sixth pandemic, another epidemic occurred in Sulawezi, Indonesia. This was declared as the 7th pandemic and was caused by the El Tor biotype of VC O1.

The El Tor biotype of VC is named for a Hajj quarantine station in Egypt where it was isolated from an asymptomatic pilgrim early in the twentieth century.

### *Vibrio cholerae*

*Vibrio cholerae* bacilli are gram-negative, curved and motile bacilli that are indistinguishable morphologically from the other enteric organisms.

- An important characteristic of all vibrios is their exacting growth requirement for salt. The pathogenic *Vibrio* is divided into two major groups; **halophilic** and **non-halophilic**. The **non-halophilic** species consist of ***V. cholerae*** and ***V. mimicus***, and will grow on routine media without salt.
- The **halophilic** species require salt (***V. para-haemolyticus, V. vulnificus, V. fluvialis, V. alginolyticus***) require salt supplement. All species (halophilic and non-halophilic) grow in the presence of higher salt (6%) concentration.

## Growth Requirements

- VC grows well on blood agar and MacConkey agar, as non-lactose fermenters.
- Selective media for the isolation of the organism include bile salt agar **(BSA)**, thiosulphate citrate bile salt sucrose agar **(TCBS)** and gelatin taurocholate thiosulphate agar **(GTTA)**.
- The colonies growing on TCBS can be divided into 2 groups based on the utilization of sucrose. The *Vibrio* that utilize sucrose produce yellow colonies (*V. cholerae* and *V. alginolyticus*) while non-sucrose utilizers give green colonies (*V. para-haemolyticus* and *V. vulnificus*).

## Virulence and Pathogenicity

### *Enterotoxin*

**Cholera toxin** is the most virulent determinant of VC. It is a polymeric protein that consists of two major components—A (active) and B (binding) region. These are encoded by ctxA and ctxB genes.

'A' region exhibits biological activity. The toxin acts by increasing the cAMP leading to protein kinase activation. This leads to altered ion transport and diarrhoeal disease. Increase in cAMP leads to sodium and chloride secretion and decreased sodium and potassium absorption. This causes loss of sodium and potassium in the intestines and inability to maintain isotonicity of intestinal fluids.

'B' region acts by facilitating the binding of toxin to the intestinal cell.

Two other enterotoxins of importance are:

**zot** (zona occludens toxin) that increase the permeability of the epithelial cells.

**ace** (accessory cholera toxin) that increases fluid accumulation.

**Cep** (core encoded pilin): its role is not known.

**Tcp A** (toxin co-regulated pilus).

**A β-haemolysin** is produced by most of VC O1 El Tor strains.

**VC O139** is genetically similar to VC O1 El Tor based upon ribotyping. It also has ctxA, tcp A genes. In addition, it has a polysaccharide capsule and outer membrane proteins (omp s).

**Adhesion factors:** They adhere to the microvilli of small intestinal epithelium and secrete enzyme mucinase that helps in adherence.

## Clinical Disease

A well-defined sequence of events occurs after the ingestion of VC that culminates in the onset of copious secretory diarrhoea. The stools have a rice water consistency. Excessive loss of fluid can lead to abdominal cramps, severe dehydration, acidosis, hypokalemia and hypovolemia. If the patient survives the intense dehydration, spontaneous recovery will ensue.

## Laboratory Diagnosis

Faecal samples are the best source of isolation. They should be immediately transported but in case of a delay **Cary-Blair** or **VR (Venkataraman Ramakrishnan) medium** can be used.

**Direct detection:** A wet preparation of the stool sample is examined under the microscope. If the organisms show a **darting** (like a dart) motility, presumptive diagnosis of *Vibrio* infection can be made. Another test to improve upon the diagnosis is done by adding a drop of the antisera on the wet preparation and looking for motile organisms. If there is loss of motility, it aids in diagnosis.

Culture and isolation are the definitive methods of diagnosis.

**Culture:** VC grows on blood agar and MacConkey agar, but selective media as TCBS and BSA are used for optimal isolation from faecal sample.

**Identification:** It is done using **polyvalent antisera** for O1 antigen followed by O139 antisera. The strains that agglutinate with neither may be non-O1 non-O 139.

Serotypes that agglutinate with O1 antisera can be characterized as serotype Ogawa or Inaba monoclonal antibodies.

Strains can be further characterized into biotype Classical or El Tor using: **Chick red cell agglutination, Lysis of sheep RBCs, Susceptibility to Mukherjee Phage IV, Polymixin B susceptibility, VP test.**

O1 or O139 can be characterized by whether they produce CT toxin or not. This can be done by:

Using broth culture of the organism to induce **Outpouring of fluids in the rabbit ileal loop.**

*In tissue culture assay-*

Rounding of $Y_1$ adrenal cells

Chinese Hamster Ovary (CHO) cell elongation.

For structural genes characterization

Latex agglutination, ELISA or PCR.

## Treatment

Fluid replacement is the most important therapy even without waiting for a confirmed diagnosis. Antibiotic therapy is reserved for serious cases. The drugs of choice are Tetracycline, Chloramphenicol and Cephalosporins.

## Prevention

Three vaccines are now commercially available in some countries. These are:

| *Characteristic* | *Type* | *Route* | *Duration of protection* | *Doses* |
|---|---|---|---|---|
| Killed cholera vaccine | Killed vaccine | i.m | 3-6 months | 2, one week apart |
| Whole cell b subunit vaccine | Killed B subunit of toxin | Oral | 2 years | 3, 12 weeks apart |
| CVD 103 HgR vaccine | Live attenuated organisms | Oral | At least 6 months | Single dose |

## *V. parahaemolyticus*

It is a halophilic marine organism that requires at least 2% sodium chloride to grow. It causes food poisoning (particularly in Japan) characterized by diarrhoea.

**Virulence**

Pathogenic strains carry thermostable direct haemolysin (TDH). Other toxin includes thermostable related toxin (TRH) .

**Epidemiology**

It inhabits brackish waters and infection is acquired by ingestion of **raw or improperly cooked seafood.**

### Diagnosis

On TCBS, they produce green colonies due to non-utilization of sucrose.

On a special blood agar known as **Wagatsuma agar** (a high salt 7% blood agar containing human O or rabbit blood), they produce β-haemolysis, produce a **Kanagawa phenomenon** that is diagnostic.

### Treatment

It is a self-limiting illness and supportive therapy is only given.

## V. vulnificus

- It causes wound and systemic infections.
- It is a halophilic marine organism that in contrast to other vibrios **ferments lactose**.
- It also possesses a polysaccharide capsule (virulence factor).
- It grows in estuarine waters and infection is contracted through open wounds leading to swelling and erythema.
- It can also contaminate shellfish. Ingestion of **raw oysters** may cause disease that is similar to other infective gastroenteritis.
- It may also lead to septicaemia.

## ENTEROBACTERIACEAE

- The members of the family Enterobacteriaceae are gram-negative, non-sporing, capsulated or non-capsulated bacilli that are either motile by means of peritrichate flagella or are non-motile.
- They are aerobic or facultative anaerobes that grow on ordinary media and ferment glucose with the formation of acid or gas or both.
- They are oxidase negative, catalase positive (except *Shigella dysenteriae* type 1) and reduce nitrates to nitire (except some strains of Erwinia and Yersinia).
- Enterobacteria are part of the normal intestinal flora or may cause gastrointestinal disturbances, but some bacteria of this genus exist in the environment.

## Classification

The family Enterobacteriaceae has been divided into 8 tribes (Ewing, 1986) on the basis of their biochemical characters.

These include:

| *Tribe* | | *Genus/genera* |
|---|---|---|
| I | *Escherichieae* | *Escherichia, Shigella* |
| II | *Edwardsielleae* | *Edwardsiella* |
| III | *Salmonelleae* | *Salmonella* |
| IV | *Citrobactereae* | *Citrobacter* |
| V | *Klebsielleae* | *Klebsiella, Enterobacter, Serratia, Haffnia.* |
| VI | *Proteae* | *Proteus, Morganella, Providencia* |
| VII | *Yersinieae* | *Yersinia* |
| VIII | *Erwinieae* | *Erwinia* |

## General Characters

- The property of lactose fermentation is of great importance in the identification of enterobacteriaceae from clinical samples.
- The specimen is plated on a medium containing lactose and neutral red indicator-**MacConkey agar.** The organisms that ferment lactose form acid which causes a pH change and turns the indicator red. Hence, colonies of **lactose fermenting (LF) organisms appear pink** while **non-lactose fermenters (NLF) remain pale.**

Other biochemical properties used in classification include:

| *Test* | *Escherichieae* | *Salmonelleae* | *Klebsielleae* | *Proteae* |
|---|---|---|---|---|
| Indole | + or - | - | - | + or - |
| MR | + | + | + or - | + |
| VP | - | - | + | - |
| Citrate | - | + | + | + or - |
| Urease | - | - | - | + |
| $H_2S$ production | - | + | - | + |
| PPA | - | - | - | + |

### Escherichia

- *E. coli* and certain related bacteria *(Klebsiella, Enterobacter, Citrobacter)* form the group known as *coliforms*.
- These are gram-negative non-sporing, non-capsulated, bacilli that are mainly motile by peritrichate flagella.
- Most of the strains have fimbriae (type I).
- It grows on ordinary media like nutrient agar, blood agar and form LF colonies on MacConkey agar.
- The biochemical reaction comprises $I_+M_+V_-C_-$ reaction that comprises (Indole, MR, VP and Citrate).

## Antigenic Structure

*E. coli* possesses 4 types of antigens:

1. **H antigen-** (flagellar antigen, from the German word **'hauch'** meaning breath). 75 antigens have been characterized. All of them are usually monophasic, and are rarely diphasic. H antigen is determined by **slide or tube agglutination.**
2. **O antigen-** (somatic antigen, from the German word **'ohne hauch'** meaning without breath). These are heat stable LPS antigen of cell wall. There are 173 antigens.
3. **K antigen-** (from the German word **'kapsel'**). These are associated with polysaccharide capsule that cause O inagglutinability.
4. **F antigen-** (fimbrial antigen). They are thermolabile proteins which are important virulence factors and have a possible role in UTI and diarrhoea (e.g. K88, L99 and colonization factor antigens). Most *E. coli* produce type 1 fimbriae.

On the basis of O antigen, *E. coli* is subdivided into a number of O groups, which are divided into subgroups on the basis of K antigen that includes strains with different H antigens.

Thus a strain of *E. coli* is recorded as O126: H27: K12.

## Virulence Factors

**Adhesion factors:** Many strains of *E. coli* develop the ability to colonize epithelial lining of the gastrointestinal and urinary tract.

Strains of *E. coli* involved in **lower UTI** have **specific O antigens** that allow adhesion to bladder epithelium.

Strains of *E. coli* involved in **upper UTI** have **P fimbrial antigens** that allow adhesion to the epithelia of the calyx and collecting ducts.

**Endotoxin (LPS):** It is found in the cell wall of all Enterobacteriaceae and has a role in toxigenicity.

**Enterotoxins:** Enterotoxigenic strain of *E. coli* (ETEC) produces 2 types of enterotoxins.

1. (a). **Heat labile toxins (LT-I and LT-II):** These are closely related to cholera toxin. They are plasmid mediated with 2 subunits- A (active) and B (binding). B subunit binds to $Gm_1$ ganglioside of epithelial cells and A subunit is released. It causes NAD dependent activation of adenylate cyclase, stimulating cAMP, which decreases sodium and chloride absorption and results in loss of water, sodium and chloride-leads to profuse diarrhoea.

   (b). **Heat stable toxins (ST):** These plasmid encoded toxins lead to guanylate cyclase activation leading to formation of cGMP within the epithelial cells. This leads to decreased co-transport of NaCl across the intestinal wall.

2. **Verocytotoxin (VT):** It is produced by enterohaemorrhagic *E. coli* (EHEC, VTEC). It is also known as Shiga-like toxin (SLT) as it is similar to Shiga toxin produced by *Sh. dysenteriae* serotype 1.

There are 2 types of VT—VT1 and VT2. (VT1 is neutralized by antisera to Shiga toxin).

The toxin consists of 2 subunits: A and B. It acts by inhibition of protein synthesis and cause mucosal damage.

**Capsule**: The K1 strain of *E.coli,* involved in 80% cases of neonatal meningitis has an antiphagocytic sialic acid capsule.

**Pathogenesis and clinical disease**

Virulent strains of *E. coli* predominantly cause gastroenteritis, UTI, pyogenic infection, septicaemia and neonatal meningitis.

## UTI

*E. coli* are the commonest organism causing UTI. There are certain strains called **nephritogenic** strains (01, 02, 04, 06, and 018) that cause UTI. In addition to host factors (age, sex, sexual activity, pregnancy, calculi and congenital abnormalities) presence of **P fimbriae** on the surface of *E. coli* mediate adherence of the organism to the uroepithelial cells. The receptor is part of P blood group antigen.

The bacteria gain access to the urinary tract by ascending or haematogenous route (more by the ascending route from faecal flora).

**Diarrhoea and dysentery:** There are 6 classes of **enterovirulent (or diarrhogenic) *E. coli*** that have been associated with gastroenteritis. They produce diarrhoea with different pathogenic mechanisms.

| *Type of strain* | *Mechanism of action* | *Type of diarrhoea* | *Method of detection* |
|---|---|---|---|
| **Enteropathogenic *E. coli* (EPEC)** | EPEC adhere to human intestinal epithelium and produce **attaching and effacing** lesions that lead to dissolution of brush border and destruction of microvilli. | Particularly in tropical countries. Characterized by profuse watery diarrhoea of varying severity and persistence. Important cause of infantile gastroenteritis | Fluorescence actin staining (FAS). HeP-2 or HeLa cell culture- show localized adherence. PCR for gene identification. |

*Contd*

*Contd.*

| | | | | | |
|---|---|---|---|---|---|
| **Entero-toxigenic *E. coli* (ETEC)** | Production of toxin. | Produces Traveller's diarrhoea. | **Ligated rabbit loop** | **LT** | **ST** |
| | | | Read at 6 hrs. | +/- | + |
| | | Common cause of dehydrating diarrhoea in children in developing countries (resembles secretory diarrhoea caused by *V. cholerae.*) | Read at 18 hrs | + | – |
| | | | **Infant mouse intragas-tric assay** | – | + |
| | | | **Adult rabbit skin (vasc perm. factor)** | + | – |
| | | | **CHO elongation** | + | – |
| | | | **$Y_1$ mouse adrenal rounding** | + | – |
| | | | **Other newer tests** EIA, LA, immuno-diffusion (BIKEN), Probes and PCR. | | |
| **Entero-invasive *E. coli* (EIEC)** | Invade the intestinal epithelium. (It does not produce Shiga toxin.) | Produces an illness (dysentery) similar to that caused by Shigella | **Sereny test-** test organism is instilled in the conjunctival sac of guinea pig- after 72 hours- keratocon-junctivitis (invasiveness). **HeLa and HeP-2cells-** for invasiveness. **PCR-** for gene identification. | | |
| **Verocyto-toxin produc-ing *E. coli* (VTEC)** | Produces a cytotoxin closely related to Shiga toxin, called Shiga-like toxin (SLT). | Cause hae-morrhagic colitis. Patient develops blood stained diarrhoea with or without | **Enterotoxic in rabbit ileal loop. Verocell culture-** cytotoxin production in HeLa cells. Latex coagglutination. **PCR for gene identification.** | | |

*Contd.*

*Contd.*

| | | | |
|---|---|---|---|
| | | abdominal pain. Also causes **Haemolytic uraemic syndrome (HUS)*.** | |
| **Diffusely adherent *E. coli* (DAEC)** | Belongs to classical EPEC serogroup, except that they show diffuse adherence in HeLa cell assay. | Its role as a diarrhoea-genic agent is contro-versial but cases have been reported from Bangladesh. | **HeLa cells**- diffuse adherence. **FAS stain**-negative unlike EPEC. |
| **Entero-aggrega-tive *E coli* (EAggEC)** | Produces a toxin called EAST (enteroaggre-gatory heat stable toxin) that induces fluid secretion. Adhesion factors. | Bloody or protracted infantile diarrhoea | **Hep-2 cells**-stacked brick like adherence. |

* HUS—It is characterized by acute renal failure, microangiopathic haemolytic anaemia and thrombocytopenia.

**Other infections:** They include pyogenic infections as wound infection and neonatal meningitis.

## Epidemiology

The transmission of *E. coli* as diarrhoeagenic agent usually occurs by faeco-oral route. Contamination of food can cause severe gastroenteritis (e.g O157: H7).

In case of UTI, *E. coli* that is endogenous in the perineum contaminates the urinary tract. In women, it is associated with sexual activity—**honeymoon cystitis.**

***Other important uses of E. coli***

*E. coli* has been used as an important indicator of faecal contamination of water samples.

The standard tests used for water bacteriology are:

**Total coliform count (presumptive count):** It is called presumptive because reaction observed may be due to presence of other organisms. It is done using double or single strength MacConkey broth with indicators.

The presumptive coliform count/ 100 ml is determined on the basis of acid and gas production in the tubes. This is done using a probability table, called McCardy's table.

The results are interpreted as:

| *Count/100 ml* | *Interpretation* |
|---|---|
| 0 | Excellent |
| 1-3 | Satisfactory |
| 4-10 | Suspicious |
| >10 | Unsatisfactory |

Other tests are—faecal coliform count and confirmed *E. coli* count.

**Eijkman test** is done for true coliform count.

Faecal streptococci and *Clostridium. perfringens* are other indicators of faecal contamination.

## Laboratory Diagnosis

### UTI

**Urine:** The normal voided urine contains urethral commensals as contaminants. Hence, collection of sterile sample is important-**mid-stream urine** is collected (clear catch). According to Kass, active bacterial infection of the urinary tract occurs when a count exceeds $10^5$ organisms/ml (denotes **significant bacteruria).** A count less than $10^4$ organisms/ml denote contamination from urethral flora.

**Direct examinations:** Microscopic examination shows increased number of polymorphs in urine-**pyuria**, which indicates UTI.

Significant pus cells seen in urine samples are:

**Uncentifuged urine:** 1 leucocyte/7 HPF in wet film corresponds to $10^4$ pus cells/ml- larger than this signifies pyuria.

**Centrifuged urine:** >3 pus cells/HPF.

### Culture

Measured quantity of urine (.004 ml), which is 1/250 ml, is inoculated onto the media (blood agar and McConkey agar) with a standardized loop (internal diameter 3.26 mm).
The number of colonies that appear on the media after overnight incubation at 37°C are counted and multiplied by 250 to find the number of organisms/ml of the urine sample. A count $>10^5$ signifies infection.

### Diarrhoea and Dysentery

The pathogen isolated from the sample that is inoculated on MacConkey and selective media are confirmed by biochemical analysis.

For detection of EPEC, colonies (at least 10 isolated colonies) are emulsified in saline on a slide and tested by agglutination with polyvalent and monovalent antisera against enteropathogenic serogroups.

### Treatment

**Rehydration** with electrolyte-rich fluids is essential when diarrhoea is profuse.

**Antibiotic therapy** is usually not indicated in *E. coli* diarrhoea except in infants, debilitated and in patients with extraintestinal infections

Trimethoprim-sulphamethoxazole is given in UTI due to *E. coli*.

A combination of ampicillin and cefotaxime is given in neonatal meningitis while in sepsis parenteral antibiotics as third generation cephalosporin with or without aminoglycoside combination are administered.

### *Shigella*

It consists of non-motile, non-sporing, non-capsulated gram-negative bacilli that do not produce gas from carbohydrates and do not ferment lactose readily on MacConkey agar.

The organisms of the genus *Shigella* cause bacillary dysentery in man which is characterized by loose motions mixed with blood and mucous.

## Classification and Antigenic Structure

On the basis of somatic O antigen and biochemical reactions, *Shigella* species have been subdivided into 4 groups.

**Group A:** It consists of *Sh. dysenteriae* which has been divided into 12 serotypes. This group, unlike other groups does not form gas from mannitol.

**Group B:** It consists of *Sh. flexneri*, which is the most complex antigenically. It is subdivided into 6 serotypes and several subtypes 1a, 1b 2a, 2b, 3a, 3b, 3c, 4a, 4b, 5a, 5b. In addition there are 2 antigenic variants called X and Y.

Serotype 6 has 3 biotypes: 88, Newcastle and Manchester.

**Group C:** It consists of *Sh. boydii* which has 18 serotypes.

**Group D:** It consists of *Sh. sonnei.* It is antigenically homogenous but undergoes antigenic variation, referred to as phase variation. There are 2 phases—I and II.

## Biochemical Reactions of the Group

- All groups form acid from glucose and other sugars except *Sh. dysenteriae,* which does not ferment mannitol.
- *Sh. dysenteriae* serotype 1, *Sh. flexneri* serotype 6 and *Sh. sonnei* are Indole negative.
- *Sh. sonnei* is a late lactose fermenter, while others are non-lactose fermenters.
- Enterobacteria are catalase positive except *Sh. dysenteriae* serotype 1 and some other strains of *Sh. flexneri* serotype 4a.

*Shigella* is non-motile and does not produce H flagella.

Adequate biochemical testing is necessary to identify *Shigella* strains adequately.

## Virulence and Pathogenicity

Invasive and toxigenic properties are the main virulence factors in *Shigella* strain but the exact role of the toxins is yet to be defined.

Plasmid and chromosomally encoded virulence factors act synergistically to determine the pathogenicity of *Shigella* species. They cause:

- Attachment to host cell.
- Invasion of cells and intercellular spread.

**Endotoxin:** It is released after autolysis. It irritates the intestinal wall and cause diarrhoea.

**Exotoxin:** *Sh. dysenteriae* serotype 1 produces a powerful cytotoxin, which is active on Vero cells and is known as **Shiga toxin**. It has 2 subunits: A (active) and B (binding). It acts by inhibiting protein synthesis.

*Shigella* after ingestion, multiply in the gut lumen after adhering to the epithelial cells. They then spread laterally into adjacent cells and deep in lamina propria. In severe cases, inflammatory reaction develops leading to necrotic patches, which slough off leaving ulcers.

## Clinical Disease

Members of the genus *Shigella* produce bacillary dysentery, which is characterized by diarrhoea in which stools contain blood and mucus. It is also associated with heavy inflammation of the colonic mucosa.

It rarely causes bacteremia or systemic infection except in immunocompromised.

Extraintestinal complications include reactive arthritis, neurological complications or **HUS** due to damage by Shiga toxin (especially by *Sh. dysenteriae* serotype 1).

## Epidemiology

*Shigella* has no animal reservoir and is a human disease. It is transmitted by faeco-oral route.

Infectious dose is as low as 10-200 organisms to induce infection.

In India, *Sh. flexneri* is the predominant causative of dysentery while in US, *Sh. sonnei* is more common.

## Laboratory Diagnosis

Shigella can be isolated from faecal sample or rectal swab.

In case of delay, sample can be transferred in **buffered glycerol saline.**

**Direct stool examination:** A large number of RBCs and polymorphonuclear cells can be seen and the background shows non-motile bacilli **(dead background).** It is important to differentiate bacillary dysentery from dysentery due to *Entamoeba histolytica.*

**Culture:** Sample is inoculated on MacConkey agar and DCA. It gives NLF colonies on MacConkey aga. Enrichment of stool samples can be done in **Selenite F broth** and gram-negative broth.

Selective media as xylose lysine deoxycholate **(XLD)** can be used to differentiate between *Salmonella* and *Shigella.*

The diagnosis is confirmed by motility and bio-chemical tests.

Serological typing is done with species-specific and type-specific antisera.

## Treatment

Most cases are self-limiting. Fluid and electrolyte replacement are the best regimen.

Antibiotics are not required and are given to very young, aged and debilitated to shorten the disease duration. The drugs of choice are Ampicillin, Co-trimoxazole, Tetracycline and Ciprofloxacin.

Multiple drug resistance to *Shigella* was first discovered in Japan in 1950's.

## Proteae

The tribe Proteae comprises three genera: **Proteus, Morganella** and **Providencia.**

They have one biochemical character that distinguishes them from all the other members of Enterobacteriaceae the ability to deaminate oxidatively certain amino acids to the corresponding ketoacids and ammonia. This is tested by growing the organism in a medium containing phenylalanine, from which phenylpyruvic acid is formed **(PPA test).**

### *Proteus*

These are gram-negative coccobacilli, which are actively motile with peritrichate flagella. They give a characteristic spreading growth **(swarming)** on appropriate solid media.

It can grow on ordinary media as nutrient agar on which swarming can be seen.

It emits a characteristic putrefactive **(fishy or seminal)** odour.

It grows on blood agar and shows NLF colonies on MacConkey agar.

## Swarming

This is a feature of *Proteus* in which a group of cells at the edge of a developing microcolony migrate to an uninoculated area of the medium.

*Swarming can be:*

**Continuous:** appear as a uniform film of growth extending over whole plate.

**Discontinuous:** series of concentric circles of growth around the point of inoculation.

*Swarming can be inhibited by:*

1. Increasing the concentration of agar in the medium from 1-2% to 6%.
2. Incorporating chloral hydrate (1 in 500), sodium azide (1 in 500), .1% boric acid, bile salt or other surface active agents.

3. By using **CLED agar** (cysteine electrolyte deficient agar).

**Diene's phenomenon:** When 2 identical strains of *Proteus* are inoculated at different points of the same culture plate, the resulting swarms of growth coalesce without signs of demarcation. However, when 2 different strains are inoculated, they remain separated by a narrow furrow. This is the Diene's phenomenon.

## Classification

Genus *Proteus* has 4 species—*Pr. mirabilis, Pr. vulgaris, Pr. myxofaciens and Pr. penneri.*

## Antigenic Structure

Motile strains possess O (somatic) and H (flagellar) antigen.

The O antigen of non-motile *Proteus* strains OX19, OX2 of *Pr. vulgaris* serotype 1 and 2 and OXK of *Pr. mirabilis* serotype 2 is shared by some rickettsiae. This is the basis of **Weil-Felix reaction** for the diagnosis of some rickettsial diseases.

## Virulence and Pathogenesis

*Proteus* is the second most common cause of UTI after *E. coli.*

The virulence factors include:

| *Virulence factor* | *Mechanism of action* |
|---|---|
| **Urease** | It hydrolyses urea in urine to ammonia and $CO_2$ which provide the bacteria with a source of $N_2$ for growth in urine.<br>Leads to alkalinization of urine, resulting in precipitation of calcium and magnesium ions to form struvite stones. |
| **Haemolysin** | Destruction of renal proximal tubular epithelial cells.<br>Promotes invasion. |
| **Fimbriae** | Help in attachment. |
| **Motility and swarming** | Help in spread of infection. |
| **Proteinase** | Promotes invasion. |

## Clinical Disease

The commonest site of *Proteus* infection is the urinary tract and *Pr. mirabilis* is the most commonly implicated.

*Pr. vulgaris* is recovered from immuno-compromised patients.

Other infections include wound infection, bedsores, osteomyelitis, infection of the umbilical stump, bacteraemia and meningitis.

## Laboratory Diagnosis

*Proteus* as a cause of UTI or other infections can be confirmed by isolation and culture from urine samples.

The pathogenic species can be further confirmed by biochemical tests.

Major differences between the 2 most commonly isolated organisms are:

| *Test* | *Pr. mirabilis* | *Pr. vulgaris* |
|---|---|---|
| Indole | – | + |
| $H_2S$ production | + | + |
| Urease | + | + |
| Acid from maltose | – | + |

### *Providencia*

These are motile organisms that swarm on nutrient agar and emit a fruity odor.

*P. stuartii* and *P. rettgeri* may cause hospital associated UTI or burn infection.

### *Morganella*

It has only one species: *M. morganii.*

They are motile and do not swarm on solid nutrient agar.

It has been isolated from diarrhoeic human stools but its role as a causative of enteritis is not yet established.

## Treatment

UTI by the members of the tribe can be treated by Benzyl penicillin and ampicillin.

In cases of resistance, newer Cephalosporins and Aminoglycosides are administered.

### *Klebsiella*

These are gram-negative, non-sporing, non-motile bacilli. Freshly isolated strains possess a well-defined polysaccharide capsule.

### Classification

*K. pneumoniae* is the type species which is further subdivided into 4 species—*K. pneumoniae* subsp *aerogenes* (also known as *K. oxytoca,* most frequently encountered), subsp *ozaenae, pneumoniae* and *rhinoscleromatis.*

It grows on ordinary media and gives large **mucoid colonies** on MacConkey agar.

### Antigenic Structure

It possesses O antigens and K (capsular) antigens. Typing can be done using bacteriocin **(Klebocin typing)** and phage typing.

### Pathogenesis and Clinical Disease

***K. pneumoniae* subsp *aerogenes*** can cause bronchopneumonia and multiple abscess formation in the lungs that can be associated with septicaemia. Other infections include nosocomial UTI, wound and burn infections, meningitis and diarrhoea.

***K. pneumoniae* subsp *ozaenae*** causes atrophic rhinitis—ozaenae-purulent infection of nasal mucous membrane.

***K. pneumoniae* subsp *pneumoniae*** causes pneumonia in immunocompromised and diabetic individuals.

***K. pneumoniae* subsp *rhinoscleromatis*** causes granulomatous disease called **rhinoscleroma** in upper respiratory tract.

## Laboratory Diagnosis

The diagnosis is based upon the isolation of the organism in culture.

It grows on ordinary media and produces very mucoid LF colonies on MacConkey agar. Freshly isolated strains have a capsule.

Further confirmation is done by biochemical testing and klebocin typing.

## Klebocin Typing

This test is based on the principal of identification of bacteriocins produced by certain strains of *Klebsiella* which are inhibitory to the other strains of the same species.

This test helps in tracing out the source of infection in epidemic caused by a particular strain.

The test stain is steaked on a plate of nutrient agar and incubated for growth overnight. When the growth appears it is scraped off, using a glass rod and exposure of the remaining colonies to chloroform. The klebocin produced from these colonies has already diffused into the media.

After removal of the test strain, some indicator strains with known klebocin type are plated perpendicular to the original strains and incubate overnight.

The pattern in which certain indicator strains are inhibited while others are not give the klebocin type of the test strain.

## Treatment

The antibiotics of choice for treatment are Trimethoprim, Nitrofurantoin and Cephalosporins.

### *Salmonella*

*Salmonella* are gram-negative, facultative anaerobic bacilli that are motile with peritrichate flagella.

These bacilli parasitize the intestine of man, causing enteric fever, gastroenteritis and septicaemia.

## Classification

The genus *Salmonella* consists of 2 species: ***S. enterica* and *S. bongori.***

There are 6 subspecies of *S. enterica,* the most important of which is *S. enterica* subsp *enterica* (subsp1) which includes the typhoid and paratyphoid serotypes.

Currently there are 2399 serotypes. All the serotypes of *Salmonella* belong to 7 DNA-hybridization subspecies: *S. enterica* subsp. *enterica, salamae, arizonae, diarizonae, houtenae, bongori* and *indica.*

## General Characters

- They are non-sporing, non-capsulated organisms. Most strains are motile with peritrichate flagella **except S. gallinarum and S. pullorum** which are non-motile.
- *Salmonella* grow on ordinary media as nutrient agar, blood agar and MacConkey agar to form **NLF colonies.** It also grows on DCA agar.
- Selective medium for its isolation is **Wilson and Blair brilliant green bismuth sulphite agar medium** (*S. typhi* and paratyphi B form black colonies). Brilliant green is inhibitory to other commensal enterobacteria and sulphite is reduced to sulphide, producing $H_2S$ that gives the colonies black metallic sheen.
- Other selective media include **xylose lysine deoxycholate XLD) agar, Salmonella-Shigella agar.**
- **Enrichment broths** are used for better isolation of *Salmonella* from stool samples. They include **tetrathionate broth, Selenite F and gram-negative broth.**
- They ferment glucose with production of acid and gas.
- The biochemical reactions are $I_{-} M_{+} V_{-} C_{+ \text{ or } -}$ (Citrate is positive in all except *S. typhi and S. paratyphi A*).

- $H_2S$ is produced by all except *S. paratyphi A.*

**Antigenic structure**

There are 3 main types of antigens:

1. O antigen- polysaccharide antigen.
2. H antigen.
3. Surface antigens, of which Vi antigen of *S. typhi* is the most important.

**O antigen:** The somatic O antigen is heat stable polysaccharide antigen, detected by agglutination and are given Arabic numerals.

**H antigen:** These are heat and alcohol labile. Heating at 100°C for 30 minutes detaches all the flagella.

In most *Salmonella*, H antigen exists in 2 phases.

**Phase 1 antigens** are serotype-specific. These are designated by small letters a to z, (except j) and then $z_1$, $z_2$ ...

**Phase 2 antigens** are widely shared and non-specific. These are designated by Arabic numerals (1-12).

There are certain strains that possess both the phases-**diphasic.**

*S. typhi,* paratyphi A and enteritidis are monophasic.

**Surface antigens**

**Vi antigen:** These are surface polysaccharide antigens, that inhibit agglutinability of the organism by O antisera. The Vi antigen of *S. typhi* is the most important pathogenically.

It is destroyed by heating the bacteria at 100°C for 1 hour.

**M antigen:** This is loose extracellular polysaccharide in *S. paratyphi B.*

**F antigens:** These are fimbrial antigens which *Salmonella* share with certain other organisms.

## Antigenic Cariation

Various *Salmonella* antigens undergo phenotypic and genotypic variation. These are:

1. **OH-O variation:** There is conversion from flagellar *Salmonella* (OH) to non-flagellar *Salmonella* (O). When flagellar *Salmonella* are cultivated on phenol (1: 800) containing agar, flagella are inhibited and O forms result.
2. **V-W variation:** All fresh isolates of *S. typhi* have Vi antigen that masks the O antigen and makes the bacilli inagglutinable. These strains agglutinate with Vi antisera and not O antisera. Vi antigen is lost on repeated subculture. This produces the W form which agglutinates with O antisera but not Vi antisera.
3. **S-R variation:** Smooth to rough variation occurs due to loss of O antigen and virulence of the strain.
4. **Variation in Vi antigen:** It is due to lysogenization with some phages that lead to alteration in serotype.
5. **Phase variation in H antigen: Cragie tube** method can be used to obtain specific phase of H antigen.

**Kauffman-White scheme of classification of *Salmonella***

This divides *Salmonella* into different O serogroups, each of which contains a number of serotypes possessing a common O antigen not found in other serotypes. These serogroups are in Arabic numerals.

The antigenic structure of a *Salmonella* serotype is expressed as an antigenic formula which has 3 parts describing the O antigen, phase 1 H antigen and phase 2 H antigen. This can be better understood in the table below:

Antigenic formulae of some important serogroups and serotypes by Kauffman-White scheme.

| *Serogroups* | | *Serotype* | *O Ags (&Vi)* | *H Ag* | |
|---|---|---|---|---|---|
| **New** | **Old** | | | **Phase 1** | **Phase 2** |
| 2 | (A) | *S. paratyphi* A | 1, 2, 12 | a | – |
| 4 | (B) | *S. paratyphi* B | 1, 4, 5, 12 | b | 1,2 |
| 7 | ($C_1$) | *S. paratyphi* C | 6, 7, (Vi) | c | 1, 5 |
| 9 | (D) | *S. typhi* | 1, 9,12 (Vi) | d | – |

Virulence and pathogenicity

| *Factors* | *Role in virulence* |
|---|---|
| Endotoxin | *Salmonella* envelope contains LPS with an antigenic polysaccharide (O Ag). |
| Invasions | Proteins that mediate adherence to and penetration into intestinal epithelial cells. |
| Factors involved in resistance to phagocytosis | *Salmonella* is a facultative intracellular organism and these help in its intracellular survival. These include—oxygen radical neutralizing factors as catalase, superoxide dismutase. |
| Ability to resist acidic pH | Help in survival. |
| Vi (virulence Ag) | Has antiphagocytic property. |

## Clinical Disease

*Salmonella* causes enteric fever, food poisoning and septicaemia.

## Enteric Fever

It is usually caused by *S. typhi* or *paratyphi* A, B and C. The incubation period is 8-15 days.

The patient presents with fever, headache, malaise, constipation, bradycardia, coated tongue, rose coloured spots on skin and abdominal discomfort. The fever shows a characteristic **stepladder** rise and lasts for 7-10 days.

Hepatosplenomegaly may develop. Patients may become carriers.

**Complications:** Intestinal perforation, haemorrhage, DIC, cholecystitis, thrombophlebitis and arthritis).

## Epidemiology

Enteric fever is acquired via faeco-oral transmission, contaminated water or food processed by asymptomatic chronic carriers. Poultry and eggs are also an important source of infection in humans.

The infectious dose varies between $10^5$- $10^9$ organisms.

### Laboratory Diagnosis

Culture and isolation of the organism are essential to confirm diagnosis.

Isolation can be done from patient's blood, faeces, urine or bone marrow.

**Direct detection:** In the early phase of disease, typhoid antigens are present in blood and urine of the patient. The various tests to detect these include:

Coagglutination (With *S. aureus* Cowan I strain).
ELISA

### Culture and Isolation

**Blood culture:** It is **positive in 90% of cases in the first week of fever,** falls to 60% in second week and is 50% in the third week.

5-10 ml of blood is collected and inoculated into blood culture bottle with 50-100 ml of 0.5% bile broth.

Large quantity of blood is required for isolation of the organism as blood is normally a sterile sample.

It is incubated at 37°C for 7 days before giving a negative report.

**Other samples**

**Clot culture:** Clot is used for culture while serum can be used for Widal test. Clot is broken up using Streptokinase.

**Faeces culture:** *Salmonella* are shed in faeces throughout the course of the disease. It can be done on MacConkey agar, DCA, Wilson and Blair media after enrichment in Sel F and tetrathionate broth.

Confirmation is done by biochemical tests and slide agglutination.

### Serology

**Widal test:** It is an agglutination test, which detects the presence of agglutinins in patient's serum against H and O antigens.

The agglutinins appear by 7-10 days of fever. **Agglutinins against H antigen appear early and last longer, while those against O antigen appear later and disappear early.**

## Interpretation

A titre of 1:100 or more for O antigen and 1:200 for H antigen is significant. A **4-fold rise in titre** in 2-week duration is significant.

False positive reactions can appear in persons vaccinated earlier with TAB vaccine, past infection or an amnestic response due to unrelated fever as malaria, viral infection, etc.

## Other Serological Tests

**Counterimmunoelectrophoresis (CIEP) for antibody detection in patient serum:** It is more sensitive and specific than Widal.

**Indirect Haemagglutination.**

**ELISA-** for antibody detection against *Salmonella* LPS.

**Solid phase RIA-** for antibody against *Salmonella* LPS.

## Treatment

Chloramphenicol has been the drug of choice, but resistance has been reported. Multidrug resistance in *S. typhi*, which is **plasmid mediated**, was first reported from India.

Other drugs for treatment include—fluoroquinolones as Norflox and Ciproflox.

Third generation cephalosporins as Ceftriaxone and Cefotaxime are also effective.

## Prevention

The vaccines used include:

| *Type* | *Content of vaccine* | *Route* | *Dose* | *Duration of immunity* |
|---|---|---|---|---|
| **Killed whole cell vaccine** | Mixture of Typhi 1000 million, Paratyphi A and B 750 million/ml. | im | 2 doses 4-6 week apart | 3 years |

*Contd.*

*Contd.*

| | | | | |
|---|---|---|---|---|
| **Live oral vaccine** | Avirulent mutant strain of S. typhi Ty21a, a stable mutant lacking the enzyme UDP-galactose. | Oral | 3 doses on alternate days | 3-5 years |
| **Recombinant vaccine** | Variant of Ty21a lacking one or several Aro genes. | — | — | Under evaluation. |
| **Purified Vi antigen vaccine** | Purified Vi antigen | im | - | Under evaluation |

**Salmonella gastroenteritis:** It is a zoonotic disease, transmitted by poultry products.

The main causative agent is *S. typhimurium*, others being *S. enteritidis*, Dublin.

It is characterized by fever, vomiting, abdominal pain and diarrhoea.

**Septicaemia:** It is characterized by suppurative lesions as osteomyelitis, deep abscess, endocarditis and meningitis.

The main causative organisms are *S. cholerasuis* and other serotypes.

## *Yersinia*

*Yersinia* belongs to the *Enterobacteriaceae* family. These are gram-negative pleomorphic coccobacilli, which exhibit bipolar staining pattern **(safety pin appearance).** They are non-motile, facultative anaerobes, catalase positive, oxidase negative and grow best at 28°C.

### Classification

The genus includes *Y. pestis,* the cause of plague (also known as **black death**), *Y. pseudotuberculosis* and *Y. enterocolitica,* important causes of human diarrhoeal diseases.

## Y. pestis

These are gram-negative pleomorphic coccobacilli which are non-motile and non-sporing. Freshly isolated organisms possess a capsule composed of a polysaccharide protein complex.

Antigenic structure and virulence

| *Factors* | *Role in disease* |
|---|---|
| Lipopolysaccharides | All the strains possess LPS that has endotoxic activity. |
| Fraction 1 glycoprotein antigen complex | The capsule contains this protein that is produced at 37°C and confers antiphagocytic properties. |
| pla | It is a protease that activates plasminogen and inactivates C3b and C5a. |
| V and W protein Ags | These are found in virulent strains. They have antiphagocytic properties and promote intracellular growth. |
| Others<br>Coagulase, pesticin 1 (bacteriocin) and fibrinolysin. | They promote the spread of infection. |

## Epidemiology

The plague bacilli have been endemic in the wild rodents of Europe and Asia. Epidemiologically, two natural cycles of plague exist. These are:

**Urban plague** occurs in cities, involving man and rodents living with him. Transmission occurs by rat fleas.

**Sylvatic plague** occurs in wild rodents (mice, squirrels and chipmunks).

Man is the accidental host and is infected by the bite of rat flea (*X cheopsis)* that causes bubonic plague.

Once patient develops pneumonic plague, transmission occurs by droplet infection.

An **outbreak of plague was reported in India in August 1994, the epicentre were Beed district (Maharashtra) and Surat city (Gujarat).**

## Clinical Disease

In man, plague occurs in three forms:

**Bubonic plague:** After an incubation period of 2-7 days, it is characterized by large lymphadenopathy in the area draining the site of flea bite. This is associated with fever, malaise and pain in the bubos. This is usually followed by bacteremia. It has a mortality rate of 50-75%.

**Septicaemic plague:** It is characterized by the presence of bacteria in blood vessels. This can manifest as haemorrhages in the skin and mucosa-hence the name black death.

**Pneumonic plague:** This occurs due to secondary spread of the bacilli in the lungs. It can be transmitted by droplet and can take up epidemic proportion. The patient presents with fever, cough with blood tinged sputum, chest pain and difficulty in breathing. It is associated with a mortality of almost 100%.

## Laboratory Diagnosis

**Direct detection:** Stain films from bubos in bubonic plague and sputum in pneumonic plague {safety pin appearance with **Wayson's stain** (bipolar staining)}.Giemsa and immunofluorescent stains are also used.

**Culture**: The specimen is plated onto blood agar and MacConkey's Agar—growth occurs in 24 hours. In broth, **stalactite pattern** of growth is seen.

**Guinea pig or white rat** inoculation is done for confirmation of diagnosis. The animal dies in 2-5 days and postmortem reveals local inflammation, oedema, regional lymphadenopathy and isolation of the organism from the organs.

**Serology:** Serum is used for retrospective diagnosis using complement fixation test or haemagglutination.

ELISA using **F1 capsular Ag** is also used.

**Treatment:** It is susceptible antibiotics as streptomycin, Chloramphenicol and Tetracycline.

*Y. enterocoitica*

These are gram-negative pleomorphic coccobacilli that are motile at 22°C.

**Antigenic structure and virulence**

It has 60 O antigenic groups and 20 flagellar (H) antigenic types.

Pathogenic serotypes produce an *E. coli* like antitoxin, which is not produced at temperatures exceeding 30°C.

Adhesions, invasions and antiphagocytic proteins also enhance virulence.

## Clinical Disease

It causes food-borne gastroenteritis and mesenteric lymphadenitis.

*Y. enterocolitica* may also cause reactive arthritis, erythema nodosum and Reiter's syndrome.

**Laboratory diagnosis**

*Y enterocolitica* can be isolated from the stool samples.

**Cold enrichment** (incubation of the sample in saline at 4°C for 1-3 weeks), increases the frequency of isolation.

**Cefsoludin-Irgasan-Novobiocin (CIN)** is a selective medium used for its isolation.

**Serology:** Antibody detection by CFT and ELISA are the other methods of diagnosis.

## Treatment

**Streptomycin, Chloramphenicol** and **Tetracycline** are the drugs of choice.

*Y. pseudotuberculosis*

- These are gram-negative, bipolar stained bacilli that are motile at 22°C (and not at 37°C)
- It is a **zoonotic** bacteria and man acquires infection through skin contact, with contaminated water or consumption of contaminated food.
- It causes **acute mesenteric lymphadenitis** in man.

- Diagnosis is by isolation from excised mesenteric lymph nodes or antibodies detection in blood.

## Other Enterobacteria

### Citrobacter

- These are motile organisms which produce Indole, are MR positive and VP negative, citrate positive and urease weakly positive.
- There are 11 species of which the most important are *C. freundii, .C koseri (C. diversus) and C. amalonaticus.*
- They grow on ordinary media as nutrient agar, blood agar, MacConkey agar and DCA.
- *C. koseri* has been responsible for several outbreaks of neonatal meningitis and brain abscess.
- *C. freundii* has been reported to cause HUS. Other infections caused by Citrobacter include UTI and cholecystitis.

### Enterobacter

- These are motile organisms which are Indole negative, MR positive, VP negative, citrate positive and produce $H_2S$.
- They can be differentiated from *Klebsiella* on the basis of motility.
- There are 2 most important species- *E. aerogenes and E. cloacae.*
- They cause opportunistic infections as UTI and wound infection.
- *Enterobacter* also causes nosocomial infections.

### Edwardsiella

- It is separated from *E. coli* on the basis of $H_2S$ production.
- *Ed. tarda* is the only species.
- They occasionally cause wound infection and are rarely isolated from diarrhoea samples,
- But its role as a causative agent of diarrhoea remains to be established.

### Hafnia

- These are motile organisms that can act as opportunistic pathogens.
- The important species is *H. alvei.*

### Serratia

- These are motile organisms that can cause opportunistic infections in neonates and the debilitated.
- The important species are *S. marcescens* (forms **red pigment**) and *S. liquefaciens.*

## NON-SPORING ANAEROBES

- They form the normal commensal flora of man and animals of oral cavity, gastrointestinal tract and genitourinary tract.
- The ratio of gut anaerobic bacteria: aerobic bacteria are 1000: 1.
- They generally act as opportunistic pathogens.

Classification of non-sporing anaerobes

| *Gram-positive bacteria* | *Gram-negative bacteria* |
|---|---|
| **Cocci** | **Cocci** |
| *Peptostreptococcus* | |
| *Peptococcus* | |
| *Sporosarcinia* | *Veillonella* |
| **Bacilli** | **Bacilli** |
| *Lactobacillus* | *Bacteroides* |
| *Bifidobacterium* | *Fusobacterium* |
| *Propionobacterium* | *Leptotricha* |
| *Actinomyces* | *Prevotella* |
| *Eubacterium* | *Porphyromonas* |

### MYCOPLASMATACEAE

- The family Mycoplasmatacae includes *Mycoplasma* and *Ureaplasma*, which are the **smallest free living bacteria.**
- They **lack a rigid cell wall**, are extremely pleomorphic and are **insensitive to cell wall active antibiotics** as penicillin and cephalosporins.

- They multiply by binary fission and do not possess flagella or pili, but exhibit **gliding motility.**
- They stain poorly with Gram stain.
- The best staining methods used are **Giemsa** and **Diene's** stain.
- The important pathogen is *M. pneumoniae.*
- *M. hominis and Ureaplasma urealyticum* also cause human infections.

## Antigenic Properties and Virulence

*M. pneumoniae* possess **two surface proteins** that mediate adhesion to the surface of ciliated mucosal epithelium.

The cell membrane bound glycolipids induce antibodies which may cross-react with brain cells leading to cell damage and neurological manifestations.

**Cold agglutinins** induced in patients with *M. pneumoniae* infection are directed against IgA determinants of RBCs leading to damage to erythocytes. The cold agglutinins are called so as they cause erythrocyte agglutination at $4^0$ C.

## Pathogenicity

*M. pneumoniae* commonly causes pneumonia, tracheobronchitis, pharyngitis, otitis media and primary atypical pneumonia (PAP). PAP is not as serious as other bacterial infection—the patient remains ambulatory **(atypical or walking pneumonia)** and is self-limiting.

## Epidemiology

The most common source of infection is inhalation of aerosoled secretions from infected individuals. They are opportunistic infectious agents.

## Laboratory Diagnosis

- These organisms cannot be stained in sputum or other samples; hence **serology and culture** are used to **confirm the diagnosis.**

- Since the organism is fastidious, they should be inoculated as soon after collection as possible. A medium widely used for its isolation is **bovine heart infusion broth (PPLO broth) and agar** with 20% horse serum and 10 % fresh yeast extract, with glucose and phenol red as pH indicators. Growth can be appreciated by **turbidity and colour change** to yellow.
- The colonies of *M. pneumoniae* appear in 1-4 weeks. They have a **fried egg appearance** and can be visualized by **Diene's stain** that gives them a dark blue centre and light blue periphery.
- **Serology/Molecular detection:** It is done for detection of antibodies and **nucleic acid.** The techniques used include direct immunofluorescence, Ag-capture ELISA, Immunoblot with monoclonal antibodies. DNA and RNA can be detected by hybridization and PCR.
- The important serological tests that help in diagnosis are:
- **Cold agglutinin:** This is characterized by agglutination of O Rh negative erythrocytes at 4°C with the antibodies present in the patients serum. A four-fold rise in titre or a single titre of ⩾ 64 is suggestive.
- **Streptococcus MG:** Serial dilution of patient's unheated sera and heat killed suspension of streptococcus MG is incubated overnight to look for agglutination. A titre of 1:20 or more is suggestive.
- **Complement fixation test:** This is for the detection of glycolipid antibodies. A four-fold rise in titre or a single titre ≥ 64 is suggestive.
- **ELISA (*M. pneumonia* specific):** For IgM, IgG and IgA antibodies.

## Treatment

They are resistant to penicillins and cephalosporins. The drugs of choice are **Tetracycline** and **Erythromycin**.

## Other Important Pathogens

### M. hominis

It causes salpingitis, tubo-ovarian abscess, pelvic inflammatory diseases in females, puerperal infection, septic arthritis, **non-gonococcal urethritis (NGU)** and pyelonephritis.

### Ureaplasma urealyticum

It causes NGU, epididymitis, vaginitis, cervicitis and puerperal fever.

Ureaplasma can be differentiated from other members by its ability to produce urease.

Tetracyclines (e.g. doxycycline) and Macrolides are the drugs of choice.

## SPIROCHAETES

### Classification

The order Spirochaetales is a heterogenous group of spiral, motile bacteria. It has two families:

**Spirochaetaceae** consists of four genera:

1. Spirochaeta
2. Treponema
3. Borrelia
4. Cristispira

**Leptospiraceae** consists of 2 genera:

1. Leptospira
2. Leptonema

### General Characters

They are long, thin, spiral rods that are motile by **endoflagella** (fine fibrils that arise from the periplasmic space in the outer membrane).

The number of endoflagella per cell is a morphological characteristic of each species—in **Treponemes** there are **3-4**, **Borrelia** has **15-20** and **Leptospira** has **1** endoflagellum.

Motility is of 3 types:

1. **Flexion and extension**

2. **Cork screw type** rotatory movement
3. **Translatory motion.**

Treponemes and Leptospira are so thin that they are seen only by **darkfield microscopy, silver impregnation stain or immunofluorescence**. Borrelia are larger and accept Giemsa stain.

## Treponemes

- These are slender organisms approximately 5-15μm long with 6-14 coils which are evenly placed at 1μm intervals.
- It is microaerophilic.
- Due to its thin structure, it cannot take up Gram's stain. In wet preparations, it can be seen by dark ground microscopy. In dried preparations, it needs to be thickened by silver impregnation methods **(Fontana's stain** for films and **Levaditi's stain** for tissue section).

## *T. pallidum and syphilis*

The pathogenic treponemes **cannot be grown** on bacteriological media and are maintained by subculture in susceptible animals. Pathogenic strains **(Nichol's strain)** of *T. pallidum* have been maintained in **rabbit testis** and in artificial maintenance medium as Nelson medium. Non-pathogenic treponemes (i.e **Reiter's strain)** can be grown **anaerobically.**

## Classification

The etiological agents of venereal and non-venereal syphilis have been recently named as subspecies of *T. pallidum.* These are:

| | |
|---|---|
| Venereal syphilis. | *T. pallidum* subspecies *pallidum* |
| *Non-venereal treponematoses* | |
| Yaws | *T. pallidum* subsp. *pertenue* |
| Endemic syphilis (also called bejel) | *T. pallidum* subsp. *endemicum* |
| Pinta | *T. carateum* |

## Antigenic Structure and Virulence

The antigenic structure of *T. pallidum* is poorly understood, as it cannot be cultured. On the basis of production of antibodies, the treponeme antigen can be divided into:

### Specific Antigens

1. **Group specific antigens:** Present in pathogenic as well as non-pathogenic preparations. The antigen used for antibody production is derived from Reiter's strain of treponemes.
2. **Species specific antigens:** These are polysaccharide in nature. *T. pallidum* is used as antigen for antibody detection.

### Non-specific Antigens

A non-specific antibody known as **reagin** antibody is seen in the blood of syphilitic patients that react with a **cardiolipin** hapten extracted from beef heart.

The virulence of the organism is related to the ability to attach to the cells and induce local inflammation.

## Epidemiology

Most cases of syphilis are transmitted by **sexual contact** and **transplacentally**, as the organisms are present in superficial genital tract.

It can also be transmitted by direct contact through mucous membrane.

## Pathogenesis and Clinical Disease

*T. pallidum* travels from the site of infection (usually skin) to the draining lymph nodes from where it reaches the bloodstream where it infects the endothelial lining causing **endarteritis.**

The incubation period is **10-90 days** and clinical manifestations fall into 4 stages:

**Primary syphilis:** It is characterized by avascular circumscribed, indurated, **painless chancre** (also known as **Hunterian chancre**) which ulcerates in the centre. This is accompanied with enlargement of the regional lymph nodes (inguinal in males and pelvic in females). The chancre is also known as the **hard chancre** to differentiate it from the soft chancre caused by *H. ducreyi.* It usually heals in 2-6 weeks, while some cases progress to secondary syphilis.

**Secondary syphilis:** It starts 2-6 months after the primary lesion heals and is due to multiplication and dissemination of treponemes in the bloodstream. The patient develops **erythematous lesions** on trunk and extremities, **mucous patches** in oropharynx and **condylomata lata** at mucocutaneous junctions. There can be systemic involvement and lymphadenopathy. The lesions heal in 4-5 years, while 13-15% progress to a latent stage and finally tertiary stage.

**Latent stage:** This stage is after the secondary lesions disappear and can be detected only by serological tests.

**Tertiary syphilis:** It is characterized by degenerative and irreversible necrotic lesions. Lesions of the heart (**aneurysm and gummata formation**) and CNS (**tabes dorsalis and general paralysis of insane**) are the most common. Few or no organisms are isolated from the lesions.

**Congenital syphilis:** *T. pallidum* can cross the placental barrier from about 16 weeks. 25% of the babies die *in utero* while 25% die during birth. Most of the surviving babies develop anomalies as IUGR, skeletal abnormalities and craniofacial anomalies.

## Laboratory Diagnosis

**Direct detection:** *T. pallidum* can be detected by **wet preparation** examination of genital and rectal lesions of primary syphilis under **dark field microscopy.** It can also be detected by **direct fluorescent antibody** staining.

Treponemes can be demonstrated in the tissues by **silver impregnation** stains.

Antigenic detection in the lesions can be done by PCR and enzyme immunoassays.

**Serology:** It is the **mainstay of diagnosis** at all the stages. The tests can be divided into **non-specific (non-treponemal) tests** and **specific (treponemal) tests.**

Non-treponemal tests

| *Test* | *Type of test* |
|---|---|
| **Wasserman test**<br>The antigen used is a **cardiolipin** antigen (extract from beef heart) with lecithin and cholesterol. | Based on CFT, detects IgG. |
| **VDRL test**<br>Most widely used **screening** test, highly **sensitive.** Positive in 70% of primary and 99% of secondary syphilis. Antibodies can be detected in 7-10 days of appearance of primary chancre. Sera have to be heated to inactivate the inhibitory substances present in it. | Slide flocculation test, detection of IgM and IgG. (Clumping under microscope taken as positive). |
| **Kahn test** | Tube flocculation test |
| **RPR test**<br>Antigen is **absorbed onto carbon particles and choline chloride** to block inhibitory substances. **No heating** of sera is required. Can be used in field areas- simple to perform and no microscope required. | Slide agglutination test<br>Screening test |

**Biological false positive (BFP) reactions:** Antibodies against cardiolipin antigen may be detected in the absence of *Treponema pallidum.* These are the biological false positive reactions. These can be **acute** reactions which appear after acute febrile illness and disappear after a short while. The **chronic** BPF reactions last for more than 6 months and are common in autoimmune diseases as SLE, leprosy, malaria, infectious mononucleosis and others.

## Treponemal Tests

A. These tests are carried out using the cultivable treponemes.

**Reiter's treponemes (*T. phagedenensis*)** is employed for group-specific antibody detection. The test used is Reiter protein complement fixation test (RPCFT). These tests are more specific than the cardiolipin test.

**B.** These are the ones in which pathogenic *T. pallidum* antigen is used. These include:

| *Test* | *Type of test* |
|---|---|
| **I. Using live *T. pallidum*** | |
| *Treponema pallidum* **immobilization (TPI) test** | It determines the ability of patient's serum to immobilize motile virulent *T. pallidum.* **Most specific test** If >50% are immobilized- it is reactive. If <20% are immobilized- it is non-reactive. If 20-50% are immobilized- doubtful. This test has the disadvantage of being expensive and it is difficult to maintain live pathogenic strains. |
| **II. Using killed *T. pallidum*** | |
| *T. pallidum* agglutination test (TPA) | In the presence of antibodies, treponemes are agglutinated. |
| *T. pallidum* immune adherence test (TPIA) | In the presence of complement, treponemes adhere to RBCs. |
| Indirect immuno-fluorescence tests<br><br>FTA (fluorescent treponemal antibody test)<br>FTA-ABS( fl. treponemal Ab absorption test)<br>**IgM FTA-ABS test** | In this test, slides fixed with *T. pallidum* are treated with patient's serum. If the serum contains antibodies, the Ag-Ab reaction is detected by adding fluorescein labelled antihuman immunoglobulin. In positive test, treponemes fluoresce. This test has a high specificity and sensitivity. They become reactive in the third week of infection- positive in 80,100 and 95% of primary, secondary and late syphilis. Specificity is 92-99%. |
| **III. Tests using *T. pallidum* extract** | |
| • T. Pallidum haemagglutination | *T. pallidum* absorbed onto RBCs is mixed with patient's serum, specific antibodies cause haemagglutination. It is easy to perform and has a high specificity and sensitivity. |
| • **Enzyme immuno-assay (EIA)** | Has sensitivity and specificity of 90 and 98%. |

## Treatment

**Penicillin** is the drug of choice. Following treatment with penicillin, some patients with active symptoms develop a reaction called the **Jarisch-Herxheimer** reaction due to the release of endotoxins.

In penicillin allergy, tetracycline or erythromycin is used.

Prognosis depends upon the result of serological tests. Earlier the treatment is started, better is the chance of seronegativity.

## Non-venereal Treponematoses

### *Endemic Syphilis (Bejel)*

- It occurs in Middle East and Africa.
- It's common in children living under poor standards of hygiene and spreads from person to person.
- The causative organism is *T. pallidum* subsp. *endemicum.*
- They present with secondary syphilis like manifestations as skin eruptions and mucous patches and can progress to tertiary syphilis.
- The diagnosis and treatment are the same as venereal syphilis.

### *Yaws*

- It is prevalent in Asia, Africa and America.
- It is caused by *T. pallidum* subsp. *pertenae.*
- The patient presents with extragenital papule that ulcerates. Secondary and tertiary manifestations may follow.
- The diagnosis and treatment are the same as venereal syphilis.

### *Pinta*

- It is common in 10-12 years old children.
- It is caused by *T. carateum.*
- It spreads by person to person contact. It also

manifests as an extragenital papule, secondary lesions may follow.

- The diagnosis and treatment are the same as venereal syphilis.

### *Treponema vincentii*

- These are 7-18 μm long spirochaetes that stain by Giemsa and Leishman stain.
- It is a normal commensal of the mouth but in predisposing conditions causes **gingivostomatitis or oropharyngitis (Vincent's angina)** which is often associated with fusiform bacillus ***Leptotricha buccalis.***

## Diagnosis

Smears stained with dilute carbol fuschin showing spirochaetes and fusiform bacilli aid in diagnosis.

### *Borrelia*

- These are large motile spirochaetes, 20-30 μm, microaerophilic with 3-10 irregular and open coils.
- *Borrelia* can be stained with aniline dyes (Wright's or Giemsa stain).
- They are easy to culture on special cell-free media and grow in **Noguchi's medium** (ascetic fluid containing rabbit kidney), **CAM of chick embryo** and **peritoneal cavity of rat or mouse.**

Two important diseases associated with *Borrelia* are:

**Relapsing fever** caused by *B. recurrentis* and other species and **Lyme's disease** caused by *B. burgdorferi.*

## Relapsing Fever

It is a febrile bacteraemia that derives its name from the fact that 3-10 recurrences are common.

It is of two types:

| | *Epidemic relapsing fever* | *Endemic relapsing fever* |
|---|---|---|
| Aetiological agent | *Borrelia recurrentis* | *Borrelia duttoni, B. hermisei* and others |
| Transmitted by | Body Louse-Pediculus corporis | Tick-Ornithodoros |
| Mode of transmission | Not by bite, but due to contamination of wounds by biting or scratching with body fluids of louse which is crushed. | Bite of the tick. |

The incubation period of fever is 3-10 days and it lasts for 3-5 days. The second attack occurs in 4-10 days. The patient presents with fever, headache, myalgia, hepatosplenomegaly and rash.

**Recurrence:** *Borrelia* undergoes antigenic variation and antigenic modulation—hence development of specific antibodies leads to termination of each episode.

## Laboratory Diagnosis

**Direct:** Blood is collected in the pyrexial period and examined under dark field microscope or by Wright's or Giemsa stain to look for spirochaetes.

Blood culture in **Noguchi's medium** and serology are important for diagnosis.

Intraperitoneal inoculation of newborn mouse or rat and isolation from the peritoneal blood within 2 days help in confirmation of diagnosis.

## Treatment

Erythromycin, Tetracycline and Penicillin are the drugs of choice. This should be supported with vector control.

## Lyme's Disease

Lyme's disease was first reported from Lyme, in Connecticut, USA.

It is caused by *Borrelia burgdorferi.* It grows on **BSK medium.**

Lyme's disease is transmitted by **ixodid tick** due to regurgitation of gut contents during meal.

The incubation period of the disease is 3-32 days. Patient develops a macule or papule with erythema that spreads centrifugally and is surrounded by induration—also known as **erythema chronicum migrans (ECM)** (Stage 1). Satellite lesions appear in 50% patients and associated symptoms of fever and regional adenopathy develop.

Patient can progress to neurological or cardiological symptoms (Stage 2) and arthritis (Stage 3).

**Diagnosis**

Clinical suspicion and awareness always aid in diagnosis.

**Direct examination:** From skin by dark field microscopy. The peripheral smears can be examined by special fluorescent antibody staining, acridine orange and Giemsa stain. The tissue specimen can be stained by silver impregnation stains.

Culture and serology (IgM-ELISA, indirect immunofluorescence and haemagglutination test).

**Treatment**

In the early stages, doxycycline is the drug of choice. In the late stages, parenteral ceftriaxone is administered.

## *Leptospira*

It consists of motile, helical, aerobic bacteria, 6-20 μm in length with hooked ends. They can be grown in enriched artificial medium, are microaerophilic and grow best at 30°C.

### Classification

Leptospira can be grouped serologically into characteristic serovars on the basis of agglutinating antigens. More than 200 serovars have been recognized. One major serological complex of leptospires known to be pathogenic is ***L. interrogans*** complex, while the other major group containing non-pathogenic leptospires is the ***L. biflexa*** complex.

There are 7 species in pathogenic group of which *L. interrogans* is the most important.

There are 3 species in non-pathogenic group of which *L. biflexa* is the most important.

### *L. interrogans*

- They are spiral bacteria, 6-20 μm long, motile with hooked ends. They are best observed with dark ground microscope, phase contrast and electron microscope.
- They stain poorly with aniline dyes but can be demonstrated with fluorescent antibody technique and silver impregnation techniques of Levaditi and Fontana.
- They are obligate aerobes that can be grown in artificial media supplemented with sterile rabbit serum or bovine serum albumin with Tween 80.

### Pathogenesis and Virulence

Leptospirosis in man can be caused by any serovars of *Leptospira*. Infection is acquired by man through contact with water, soil or vegetations **contaminated with animal urine**. They enter the body through cuts and abrasions of the skin or mucous membrane of the nose, mouth or eyes.

The organism enters the bloodstream and spreads haematogenously to the other organs and tissues.

### Clinical Disease

It has an incubation period of 1-2 weeks.

**Acute or anicteric phase:** The early symptoms are influenza like and non-specific. The patient develops severe headache, fever, nausea, vomiting and myalgia. Purpuric haemorrhages in skin and mucosa are often seen. Leptospires can be seen in the blood in the early phase.

**Icteric phase:** This is the severe form of disease. Disseminated endothelial damage and vasculitis may lead to impaired renal and hepatic functions, internal haemorrhages, meningitis, cardiovascular collapse DIC and shock. Hepatomegaly is detected in 25% of cases and is usually associated with jaundice. Kidney involvement is reflected by acute tubular necrosis and renal failure. ***L. interrogans*** **serovar** ***icterohaemorrhagiae*** produces a more severe illness known as **Weil's disease** (infectious jaundice), though the other serovars can also be associated with the disease.

## Epidemiology

*L. interrogans* are animal pathogens.

**Rats** are the most significant vector worldwide but dogs, cats and livestock can also harbour the organism.

It can spread during overcrowding due to poor sanitation (slums, post-floods) and open drainage.

In India, Andaman Islands and coastal areas are endemic for Leptospirosis.

## Diagnosis

Leptospirosis usually presents as PUO, hence diagnosis generally requires a high level of clinical awareness of its transmission, but confirmation can be achieved through demonstration of Leptospires and serological diagnosis.

**Direct detection:** Leptospires can be demonstrated **in blood or CSF by dark ground microscopy** during the first week of illness and from urine in the later course of the disease.

The **culture** can be done in **modified Korthof's** medium and examined every 3 days using dark field microscopy (DFM) for 6 weeks. Serovar identification can be done by agglutination.

**Serology:** Antibodies appear in serum at the end of first week and peak in approximately 4 weeks after which they begin to decline. The tests fall in two categories:

**Genus specific tests:** These detect leptospiral infections without indicating the serovar. The antigen is prepared from non-pathogenic **L-biflexa Patoc 1** strain. The tests can be CFT and ELISA for IgM and IgG.

**Serogroup and serovar specific tests:** These are used to demonstrate specific antibodies. **Macroscopic and microscopic agglutination tests** are used.

- **Macroscopic agglutination test:** It consists of formalin killed suspension of reference strains. The test is carried out by looking for macroscopic agglutination.
- **Microscopic agglutination test (MAT):** It consists of formalinized or living suspension of well grown cultures of reference strains and results are obtained by looking for agglutination under low power DFM.

## Treatment

Penicillin is the drug of choice. In allergic patients, Tetracycline, Streptomycin and Erythromycin are used.

## MYCOBACTERIA

- Mycobacteria are non-motile, non-sporing, aerobic or microaerophilic, straight or slightly curved rod-shaped bacteria.
- The first member of this genus to be identified was the Hansen (Leprae) bacilli by Hansen followed by the tubercle bacilli by Koch.
- Mycobacteria are **acid-alcohol fast** i.e once stained with a specific dye; the cells resist decolorization with acidified ethanol. The basis of acid-fast staining is related to the presence of **mycolic acid** in the cell wall, to the integrity of the cell and the viability of the cell. Hence, they are

difficult to stain with the aniline dyes, but once stained with **hot carbol fuschin**, they resist decolorization with dilute mineral acid and alcohol. Thus, they are referred to as acid-fast bacilli **(AFB).**

## Classification

On the basis of growth rate, the species fall under two groups—**slow growing species** require more than 7 days to form visible colonies on solid media, while **rapid growers** require fewer than 7 days. There are currently 71 species of Mycobacteria that are grouped into 2 major divisions-**rapidly growing** and **slowly growing.**

The type species is ***M. tuberculosis.***

The slowly growing species are further divided into 3 groups based on pigmentation. This is the Runyon classification.

| | |
|---|---|
| Photochromogens | Form pigment in light. |
| Photochromogens | Form pigment in dark. |
| Non-photochromogens | Do not form pigment in light or darkness. |

Most cases of human tuberculosis are caused by *M. tuberculosis,* but some are caused by *M. bovis.*

*M. africanum* includes heterogenous strains with properties intermediate between *M. tuberculosis* and *M. bovis*. Hence this causative agent of pulmonary tuberculosis is a member of **M. tuberculosis complex (M. tuberculosis, M. bovis and M. africanum).**

## M. tuberculosis

- It is a slender, straight or slightly curved rod, which is non-motile, non-sporing, non-capsulated and acid-fast.
- The tubercle bacilli stain bright red with **Zeihl Neelsen** acid-fast stain, while the tissue cells and other organisms are stained blue. The organisms

in tissue and sputum often stain irregularly and have a **beaded appearance.**

- It can also be stained by **auramine O** (fluorescent stain), which is very sensitive.

**Culture media:** Tubercle bacilli is microaerophilic and grows well on enriched culture media.

Many laboratories use a combination of broth and solid media to enhance the recovery of the organism.

**Broth:** Mycobacteria grow quickly in broth media than solid media, e.g. **Middlebrook 7H9** and **Kirshner's** medium. The problem with these media is increased chance of contamination before isolation of mycobacteria which is inhibitory to the organism.

**Solid media:** Egg based media support good growth of mycobacteria. One such medium is the **Lowenstein Jensen (LJ) medium.** This medium consists of whole egg, asparagines, some mineral salts, malachite green and glycerol which is solidified by inspissation. Malachite green inhibits the organisms other than mycobacteria and provides a colour contrast to the medium. Glycerol stimulates the growth of *M. tuberculosis* and decreases that of *M. bovis.*

*M. tuberculosis* grows well on LJ medium **(eugonic growth),** while *M. bovis* grows poorly on LJ medium (**dysgonic growth).**

**Agar based media: These** include **Middlebrook 7H10 and 7H11 agar.** They are transparent media; hence determination of minute colonies can be quicker than egg based media.

The medium is incubated for at least 6 weeks for clinical specimen and upto a total of 12 weeks.

## Cell Wall and Antigenic Structure

It consists of lipids, peptidoglycans, lipoarabinomannan, mycosides and mycolic acid. Lipids account for 60% of the cell wall weight and contribute to:

- Increased hydrophobic character of mycobacteria (they adhere to each other during growth).
- Acid fastness of the organism.

- Slow growth and formation of clumps and cords.

**Lipoarabinomannan** is structurally and functionally related to O-antigenic LPS of other bacteria. It is also responsible for biological activities of the bacteria. Mycobacteria possess two types of antigens:

Cell wall (insoluble) and cytoplasmic soluble antigens.

**Cell wall antigens:** Arabinomannan, arabinogalactan and lipoarabinomannan.

**Cytoplasmic antigens:** Membrane bound proteins, increase molecular weight carbohydrate, lipid, mycolic acid, etc. Various serological tests as ELISA, RIA and Latex agglutination are used for serodiagnosis of tuberculosis using these.

## Pathogenicity and Virulence Factors

The virulence factors for *M. tuberculosis* have not been as well defined as those for many other bacteria.

Mycobacteria characteristically survive after ingestion by macrophages and behave as facultative intracellular organisms.

The toxic substances include:

**Cord factor:** Inhibits migration of polymorphonuclear cells and hence **elicits granuloma formation**. They cause bacteria to grow in **serpentine cords.**

**Sulfatides:** Decrease phagolysosome formation and permit the organism to survive intracytoplasmically.

Though these factors are synthesized by mycobacteria, it is doubtful whether they play a major role in determining its virulence.

The mechanisms hypothesized for how the tubercle bacilli avoid being killed by macrophages include:

- Prevention of an oxidative burst in phagocytosing cells.
- Inhibition of phagosome-lysosome fusion.
- Resistance to lysosomal enzymes as lysozyme.

- Secretion of inhibitors of bactericidal agents as peroxidases or oxygen radicals.
- Escape from phagosome into the lysosome.

## Pathogenicity and Clinical Disease

*M. tuberculosis* affects one-third of the world's human population and causes 7% of all the deaths.

Protective immune reactions in tuberculosis are principally cell mediated and humoral immune response is regarded as having no protective role to play.

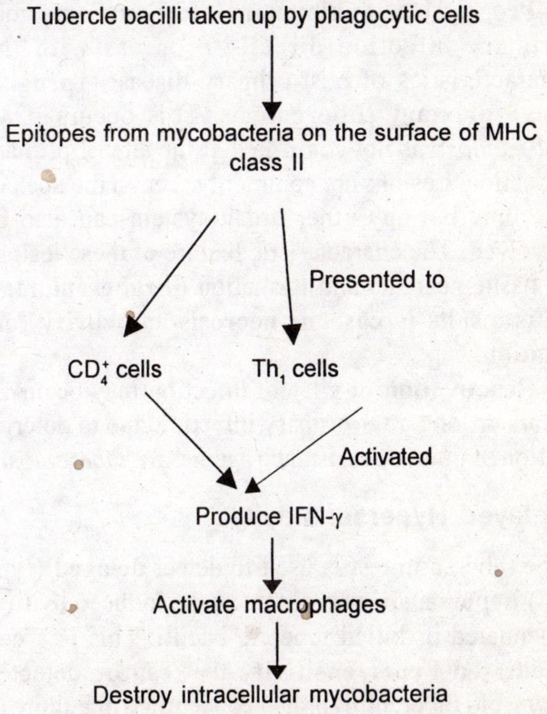


**Primary tuberculosis:** Disease occurring in a person never previously exposed to the tubercle bacilli is termed primary tuberculosis. Infection results in a focus of disease **(the Ghon's focus)** at the site of implantation of bacillus, usually the lung, along with the infected regional lymph node which is known as the **primary complex.**

The primary complex often resolves but may cause local serious complications. Haematogenous spread may occur with the implantation of tubercle bacilli in many organs. Foci developing in the endothelium of major blood vessels may rupture and give rise to **disseminated or 'miliary tuberculosis'.**

**Post-primary (secondary) tuberculosis:** It develops in previously infected persons due to endogenous reactivation of latent disease or exogenous infection. This is usually seen 5 years after primary infection.

**Progression of pulmonary infection:** Sometimes primary infection directly progress with the characteristics of post-primary disease—**progressive primary tuberculosis.** This occurs if *M. tuberculosis* is not controlled at the site of primary infection. Lesions are commonly seen in the apex of the lung but any other organ system can also be involved. The characteristic feature of these lesions is tissue necrosis and formation of **tuberculomas**. This results in **caseous necrosis** and **cavity formation.**

**Reactivation** of a latent infection may occur 20 years or long after primary infection due to deterioration of immune resistance against *M. tuberculosis.*

## Delayed Hypersensitivity

The tuberculin test is used to detect **delayed (type IV) hypersensitivity** which can be induced by live, attenuated or killed tubercle bacilli. This is a **cell mediated hypersensitivity** that can be detected using old tuberculin (boiled concentrate of culture of tubercle bacilli) and **purified protein derivative (PPD,** refined tuberculin).

**Montoux test**: 0.1 ml of PPD containing 5 IU is injected intracutaneously into the skin of the volar aspect of forearm. The site is palpated after 72 hours. Development of an area of firm induration of 10 mm or more is taken as positive, 5-9 is doubtful and <5 mm is negative. The extent of erythema is irrelevant.

1 TU is used when extreme hypersensitivity is suspected and 250 U is used only rarely, when 5 and 10 TU tests are negative.

**Heaf test:** It is done with a multiple puncture apparatus with six needles that prick 1-2 mm deep in the skin. The test is read after 72 hours. Erythema and induration around at least 4 punctures is positive.

## Uses of the Test

- To diagnose infection in infants and young children.
- To demonstrate prevalence of infection in a community.
- To select susceptibles for BCG vaccination.
- To assess the effectiveness of control measures and aid diagnosis.

**Infection is usually negative in early and advanced tuberculosis, military tuberculosis and in patients with viral infection, immunosuppressive therapy, advanced age and lymphoid malignancy.**

**False positive reaction:** Seen in patients with atypical mycobacterial infections.

## Epidemiology

An estimated 8-10 million people develop overt tuberculosis and at a given time an estimated 20 million patients have tuberculosis, of which 70-80% are in poor nations.

Low socioeconomic status and malnutrition are important predisposing factors.

Doctors, nurses and lab workers who have contact with patients are prone to develop the disease. AIDS patients are also at high risk.

The major source of infection is the open human case shedding the bacillus in the sputum.

## Laboratory Diagnosis

Lab diagnosis of tuberculosis can be established by demonstrating the bacillus in the lesions by microscopy, isolating it in culture or transmitting the infection to experimental animals.

**Specimen:** The choice of specimen is usually determined by patient's clinical presentation. The **volume** is important as the body fluids contain few organisms, submission of higher volume and more number of samples is important. Urine, sputum and gastric aspirate should be submitted for 3-5 days.

**Early morning specimen** is the best as organisms have accumulated overnight.

## Microscopy

Smears are stained by Ziehl-Neelsen technique and examined under oil immersion. AFB stains bright red against a blue background.

To be detected microscopically, there must be 50,000-100,000 bacteria/ml of sputum.

Staining with auramine O and rhodamine B and examination under fluorescent microscope is also a useful and sensitive technique.

## Concentration Methods

Mycobacteria can be concentrated and decontaminated into a small volume without inactivation. Such concentration can be used for microscopy, culture and animal inoculation. These are:

**Petroff's method** using 4% sodium hydroxide and hydrochloric acid.

Instead of alkali, homogenization can be done with treatment with dilute acids (5% oxalic acid, 3% HCl or 6% sulphuric acid), **N-acetyl cysteine with sodium hypochlorite, zephiran** and **cetrimide.**

### *Culture*

It is a sensitive method for determination of as few as 10-100 bacilli/ml in the specimen as well. Cultures are examined for growth for 4 days (for rapid growers) and at least twice weekly thereafter. A negative report is given if no growth appears after 8-12 weeks.

**Biochemical tests:** Several biochemical tests for identification of tubercle bacilli are used. These include:

| *Test* | *Result* |
|---|---|
| **Niacin test** | Human bacteria give a positive reaction, while bovine type is negative. |
| **Aryl sulfatase test** | Positive by atypical mycobacteria. |
| **Catalase peroxidase test** | Most atypical bacteria are strongly positive, tubercle bacilli is weakly positive. Tubercle bacilli and not atypical mycobacteria are peroxidase positive. Loss of catalase and peroxidase activity in tubercle bacilli is associated with the development of resistance to Isoniazid. |
| **Nitrate reduction test** | Positive for *M. tuberculosis* and negative for *M. bovis*. |

## Sensitivity Testing

After the emergence of multidrug resistance (MDR), it is essential to perform sensitivity testing on tubercle bacilli as an aid and guide to treatment.

**Absolute concentration method:** In this method, serial dilution of drug is inoculated on media and the MIC is calculated from the media with the least drug concentration that inhibits growth.

**Resistance ratio method:** Two sets of media containing graded concentration of the drug are inoculated. One set of media contains the test strain and the other set is inoculated with a strain of known sensitivity.

**Proportion method:** In this method, the number of colonies growing from a strain inoculated on a drug containing medium is compared with the colony count from same size inoculated on a drug free medium. The strain is resistant when >1% bacteria grow in the presence of the drug.

## Animal Inoculation

Guinea pig inoculation is done for diagnosis of tuberculosis.

*M. tuberculosis* is highly pathogenic for guinea pigs and non-pathogenic for rabbits, while *M. bovis* is highly pathogenic for both guinea pig and rabbits.

## Serodiagnosis

- ELISA tests using various antigens of *M. tuberculosis* and *M. bovis* for IgM, IgA and IgG.
- RIA tests have a higher sensitivity and specificity than ELISA for antigen and antibody detection.
- Latex agglutination for antibody detection.
- Improved techniques for early detection

**Radiometric methods**

**Bactec 460 TB system:** Mycobacteria are grown in a media supplemented with palmitic acid in which carbon is radiolabelled and the growth is detected by measuring the release of $^{14}CO_2$. This technique is very sensitive and rapid for isolation of mycobacteria.

**BacT/ALERT microbial detection system:** It detects $CO_2$ derived changes by a calorimetric sensor at the bottom of the bottle.

**Manual mycobacterial growth indicator tube (MGIT):** This is a rapid and easy method of growth detection based on measurement of fluorescence production by the growing bacteria.

**Non-Radiometric methods**

- ESP culture system
- Septi chek AFB system
- Luciferase technique based upon the use of mycobacteriophages.
- Other molecular methods

**Chromatographic analysis:** Gas liquid or high performance chromatography is used for analysis of fatty acids extracted from cell wall of an isolate. This helps in the identification of various species of mycobacteria.

**Nucleic acid hybridization:** This is done using nucleic acid probes based on total DNA or ribosomal DNA is used to identify several mycobacteria.

**PCR gene amplification method:** It is based upon the use of oligonucleotide primers to detect the amplification of specific nucleic acid which can be DNA or RNA based. Experience with insertion sequence 6110 based systems is doubtful. Other system used is the ROCHE AMLICOR.

This test has a **disadvantage** of lacking specificity as false positivity is high. It cannot differentiate between dead and live DNA of the organism, and hence; treated or old cases can also be detected as positive.

## Treatment

The treatment of tuberculosis involves simultaneous administration of at least two drugs to avoid resistance stains of *M. tuberculosis.* Hence, 3-4 drugs are given simultaneously.

The antitubercular drugs are **Rifampicin, Pyrazinamide, Streptomycin, Ethambutol** and **Thiacetazone.** The first four are bactericidal.

The period of treatment depends upon the type of tuberculosis and short course regimen of about 6 months with drugs as rifampicin have been found adequate in many cases.

The standard regimen recommended by WHO, 1994, for adults is known as **directly observed therapy short course (DOTS).**

It consists of:

**Two months of intensive phase with Isoniazid (H), Rifampicin (R), Pyrazinamide (P)** and **Ethambutol (E)** or **Streptomycin(S) given daily, followed by 4 months of maintenance therapy with Isoniazid and Rifampicin given thrice weekly.**

All the drugs are given under **direct supervision.**

## Immunoprophylaxis

Administration of **bacille calmette guerin (BCG),** an attenuated strain of *M. bovis,* is used as an effective vaccine. Its efficacy has always varied from 0-80%.

It does not protect against tuberculosis but prevents its complications in neonates as meningeal and military tuberculosis.

## Drug Resistance in Tuberculosis

The problem of drug resistance is on an increase in both developing and developed countries. Since early 1990's several outbreaks of **MDR TB** have been reported from different regions of the world as a consequence of inappropriate use of essential antitubercular drugs.

The mechanisms of drug resistance in *M. tuberculosis* are:

| *Drug* | *Mechanism of action* | *Genes involved in resistance* | *Mechanism of resistance* |
|---|---|---|---|
| **Isoniazid** | Inhibition of mycolic acid synthesis. | (i). Kat G (catalase-peroxidase) (ii). inhA (enoyl-ACP reductase) | Prevention of activation of INH. Overexpression of INHA allows continuation of mycolic acid synthesis. |
| **Rifampicin** | Inhibition of transcription. | rpoB (B subunit of RNA polymerase). | Mutation in rpoB prevents interaction with rifampicin. |
| **Streptomycin** | Inhibition of protein synthesis. | RPSL (ribosomal protein S12). Rrs(16SrRNA) | Mutation prevents interaction with streptomycin. |
| **Ethambutol** | Inhibition of arabinogalactan and lipoarabinomannan synthesis. | EmbAB(arabinosyl transferase) | Overexpression of gene causes continuation of arabinan biosynthesis. |
| **Pyrazinamide** | Unknown. | PcnA | Decrease in activation of the drug. |
| **Fluoroquinolones** | Inhibition of DNA gyrase. | GyrA(DNA gyrase subunit A) | Mutation in gene prevents interaction with fluoroquinolones. |

## MDR BACILLI

MDR bacilli are resistant to at least Isoniazid and Rifampicin, the main antitubercular drugs. This is the most severe form of bacterial resistance.

The various drugs used for its treatment are Aminoglycosides, Thiomides (Ethionamide), Ofloxacin, Pyrazinamide, Ethambutol and Cycloserine.

## Mycobacteria Other than Tuberculosis (MOTT)

Several species of mycobacteria other than *M. tuberculosis* can infect humans. These organisms, with the exception of *M. leprae (*which is classified separately) are generically designated MOTT, atypical mycobacteria or **nontuberculous mycobacteria (NTM).**

These organisms normally exist as saprophytes of soil and water and occasionally cause opportunistic diseases in man.

Classification of MOTT

| Type | Examples |
|---|---|
| I Photochromogens | *M. kansasii, M. marinum* |
| II Scotochromogens | *M. scrofulaceum, M. gordonae* |
| III Non-chromogens | *M. avium-intracellulare, M. xenoti,* |
| *M. ulcerans* | |
| IV Rapid growers | *M. chelonei, M. fortuitum.* |

The important NTM include:

| *Mycobacteria species* | Disease caused |
|---|---|
| ***M. kansasii*** | It can cause pulmonary disease resembling tuberculosis.<br>Rarely causes lymphadenitis, skin and soft tissue infection. |
| ***M. avium-intracellulare*** | Causes pulmonary infection in cavities in patients with cystic fibrosis or COPD or immunocompromised.<br>Causes lymphadenitis in children.<br>Disseminated infection in AIDS patients with CD4 count <50/µl. |
| ***M. scrofulaceum*** | Granulomatous cervical lymphadenitis in children. |

*Contd.*

*Contd.*

| | |
|---|---|
| | Disease syndrome resembling tuberculosis. |
| *M. abscessus* | Skin and soft tissue infection. |
| *M. chelonei* | Skin and soft tissue infection. |
| *M. fortuitum* | Skin and soft tissue infection. |
| *M. marinum* | Skin and soft tissue infection. |

All the above rarely cause disseminated infection in immunocompromised and immunosuppressed patients.

## M. leprae

It is the causative agent of leprosy **(Hansen's disease)**, a chronic mycobacterial disease, predominantly affecting the skin and peripheral nerves.

### General characteristics

Leprosy bacilli are straight or slightly curved slender bacilli.

They are less acid-fast than tubercle bacilli with ZN stain and hence 5% $H_2SO_4$ is used for decolorization after staining with carbol fuschin. The leprae bacilli are usually seen inside the cells (mainly in histiocytes) as bundles of 50 or more organisms bound together—these masses are called **globi.**

Live bacilli stain uniformly while dead bacilli appear granular or beaded.

### Cultivation

*M. leprae* **cannot be cultured** in bacterial media.

It can be maintained in the **foot pad of mice** and **9-banded armadillo** (*Dasypus novemcinctus*).

Attempts at cultivation of *M. leprae* using artificial culture media are on—one such is the Indian Cancer Research Centre (ICRC), Bombay, strain which was isolated from leprosy patient and claimed to be cultivated in human foetal spinal ganglion cell culture.

Other animals used for its propagation are Korean chipmunks, Indian pangolins and monkeys.

### Antigenic structure and virulence

The antigens include—soluble antigens (cytoplasmic) and insoluble antigens (cell wall lipid bound).

The cell wall consists of peptidoglycan, lipo-arabinomannan-B (LAM-B), mycolic acid and mycosides. A major component of the outermost layer is **phenolic glycolipid-1 (PGL-1).**

**LAM-B:** It is highly antigenic and helps in serodiagnosis.

**PGL-1:** It protects against host cell enzymes and inhibits cell-mediated immunity.

## Pathogenesis

*M. leprae* can survive and replicate in phagocytic cells. It evades host immune response by:

- Inhibiting phagocyte-lysosome fusion and escaping from phagocyte to cytoplasm.
- Inhibition of IFN-β-mediated macrophage activation.
- Resistance to oxygen radicals (by PGL-1 and LAM-B) and induction of enzymes as catalases and superoxide dismutase.

## Immune response

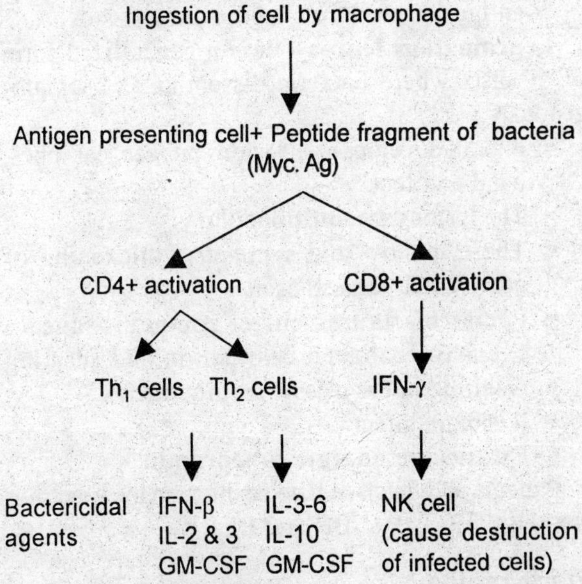

## Clinical Disease

*M. leprae* causes chronic granulomatous disease with a predilection for skin, nerves and nasal mucosa.

On the basis of clinical, histopathological and immunological findings, **Ridley** and **Jopling** introduced a scale to classify the specimen of leprosy into 5 groups:

TT BT BB BL LL

**Tuberculoid leprosy:** It is seen in patients in whom CMI is intact.

- Skin lesions are few and consist of macular patches involving face, trunk and limbs.
- There are very few AFB in the lesion-**paucibacillary disease.**
- Giant cells are abundant and lymphocytic infiltration in lesions is extensive.
- The bacilli invade local sensory nerves and gradually extend into bigger nerve trunks, leading to deformity of hands and feet.
- CMI is intact and patients **show a delayed type hypersensitivity reaction to Lepromin**, an antigen derived from lepromatous tissue.

**Lepromatous leprosy:** It is a generalized form of disease, where bacteria disseminates haematogenously.

- Patient develops skin lesions on face, ear lobes, hand and feet.
- The lesions are **multibacillary.**
- There is slow and symmetric thickening of nerves and paraesthesia.
- Facial disfigurement is common—due to extensive collagen destruction and scarring resulting in the classic **leonine facies.**
- It is more infectious.
- Patients are **anergic to lepromin.**

Patients with intermediate position on the spectrum are classified as BT, BB and BL.

## Epidemiology

Leprosy is not a very contagious disease.

Close contact with infected persons increase the risk of disease which can be transmitted by contaminated droplets.

Incubation period is extremely long- several months to 20 years.

## Laboratory Diagnosis

Diagnosis is primarily based upon clinical signs and symptoms.

## Direct Detection

Smears are made from affected parts of the skin **(slit skin smears)** and nasal mucosal membrane—these are stained by ZN method and examined under the microscope for acid-fast bacilli.

The smears are made from the areas more likely to be affected and in a patient with diffuse infiltration 5-6 different areas of the skin should be sampled.

## Animal Inoculation

Ground tissue from lepromatous nodules and nasal scrapings can be inoculated into the foot pad of mouse. It develops granuloma within 1-6 months.

Nine-banded armadillo is also susceptible—develops generalized infection with extensive multiplication of the bacilli.

## Lepromin Test

The antigens used can be of human origin (Lepromin-H) or of armadillo origin (Lepromin-A).

0.1 ml of lepromin is injected intradermally—response is seen in 2 phases.

1. **Early or Fernandez reaction**—It is characterized by a local inflammation with congestion and oedema which is >10 mm in diameter. It appears in 24-48 hours and disappears in 3-4 days.
   Histologically, it shows lymphocytic infiltration.
2. **Late or Mitsuda reaction**—A nodule appears in 3-4 weeks that may undergo necrosis and ulceration. It is a manifestation of CMI.

### Uses of the Test

- Classify lesions of leprosy, it is **positive in tuberculoid** leprosy and **negative in lepromatous** leprosy.
- **Assess prognosis** and **response to treatment.** Positive reaction indicates good prognosis and conversion to positivity is the evidence of response to treatment.
- Assess the resistance of individuals to leprosy and recruitment of persons to work in leprosy homes—lepromin positive persons are recruited as they have good CMI against the disease.

### Treatment

Multidrug therapy is recommended for the treatment of leprosy.

**Dapsone** is the most important drug.

Treatment regimen is:

| *Paucibacillary lesions (TT, BT)* | *Multibacillary lesions (BB, BL, LL)* |
|---|---|
| Dapsone 100 mg daily.<br>Rifampicin 600 mg once a month<br>Duration of treatment:<br>**6 months.** | Rifampicin 600 mg once a month.<br>Dapsone 100 mg daily<br>Clofazimine 50 mg daily<br>Duration of treatment:<br>**2 years.** |

### Control and Prophylaxis

Partial protection after administration of BCG has been reported.

Other candidate antileprosy vaccines include:

BCG+ killed *M. leprae*
ICRC bacillus
*Mycobacterium w*

Second generation vaccines—natural or recombinant vaccines, under trial.

## CHLAMYDIA

They are small **obligate intracellular** bacteria which lack the ability to synthesize ATP (use host ATP), **do not grow on artificial media** and are non-motile.

They stain poorly with Gram stain but readily with Giemsa, Casteneda, Gimenez and Macchiavella methods.

They show inclusion bodies which are basophilic in nature.

*Chlamydia* were earlier considered to be viruses due to:

- Filterability
- Ability to grow in cell free media.

They **differ from viruses** in the following properties:

- Possess both DNA and RNA.
- Have cell wall and ribosomes.
- Replicate by binary fission.
- They are susceptible to antibiotic and chemotherapy.

## Classification

The family Chlamydiaceae has a single genus Chlamydia. There are 4 species—*C. trachomatis, C. psittaci, C. pneumoniae* and *C. picorum.*

The features of the 4 species are given in the table below:

| *Characters* | *C. trachomatis* | *C. pneumoniae* | *C. psittaci* | *C. pecorum* |
|---|---|---|---|---|
| **Natural hosts** | Human, pigs, mice | Human, horses | Birds, mammals, occasionally humans | Cattle & sheep |
| **EB morphology** | Round | Round or pear-shaped | Round | Round |
| **Inclusion body** | Oval, vacuolar | Oval, dense | Variable, dense | Oval, dense |
| **Iodine staining** | Yes | No | no | No |
| **Sulphonamide sensitivity** | Yes | no | No | No |
| **No. of serovars** | At least 15 | 1 | Undefined | 3 |
| **Characteristic infection** | Oculogenital Often inapparent Intermittent shedding | Chronic respiratory tract infection | Frequent systemic pneumonia, abortion, etc. | CNS, respiratory and gut, Prolonged carriage possible. |

## Life Cycle

There are 2 morphologically distinct forms of Chlamydiae, namely elementary body (EB) and reticulate body (RB).

**Elementary body:** It is the **infectious extracellular** form.

It is 250-350 nm in diameter and is the most differentiated form.

It is responsible for spreading the infection within a host and host-host transmission.

Infection is initiated by the attachment of EB to the target cell of the host (as columnar or transitional epithelial cells).

It attaches to the surface of the cell and is phagocytosed. *Chlamydia* escapes degeneration by phagosome-lysosome fusion.

**Reticulate body:** It is the replicative, intracellular form.

It evolves from the EB 5-6 hours after penetration of the target cell.

Once differentiated, the RB begins to divide by binary fission and continues to divide for 18-24 hours.

**Inclusion bodies:** These are **intracytoplasmic** vacuoles that contain replicating organisms. They are **perinuclear** and can be visualized by conventional microscopy of infected cells.

They are basophilic in nature.

Cells infected by *C. psittaci* and *C. pneumoniae* show multiple small inclusion bodies scattered around the nucleus while cells infected by *C. trachomatis* show a single large inclusion body.

## Antigenic Structure

They possess the following antigens:

1. **Genus-specific antigens:** It is an LPS protein complex present in both RB and EB.
2. **Species-specific antigen:** MOMP (Major outer membrane protein) has species-specific epitopes and consists of 5 constant and 4 variable sequence regions.

3. **Serotype-specific antigen:** *C. trachomatis* is divided into 15 serotypes on the basis of MOMP. It possesses 3 biovars:
   1. **TRIC**-those causing Trachoma and inclusion conjunctivitis.
   2. Those causing **LGV**.
   3. Ones causing mouse pneumonitis.

## Virulence and Pathogenicity

All *Chlamydia* are highly infectious but species differ in their degree of virulence. The pathogenic mechanism is not fully understood, but their ability to replicate intracellularly and production of both exotoxins and endotoxins are believed to play major roles.

Intracellular survival seems to be associated with the ability of the RB to inhibit phagosome-lysosome fusion.

## Clinical Disease

The most important pathogen in *Chlamydia* is *C. trachomatis* which has 3 biovars and the infections caused by it are listed in the table below.

| *Biovars* | *Serotypes* | *Infections caused* |
|---|---|---|
| TRIC | A, B, Ba, C | Trachoma |
| | D-K | Non-gonococcal urethritis—urethritis (most common in males), epididymitis, cervicitis (most common in females), salpingitis, procitis. Inclusion conjunctivitis, Ophthalmia neonatorum, pneumonia in infants, abortions and stillbirth. |
| LGV | L1, L2 and L3. | Lymphogranuloma venereum. |

## Genital Infections

LGV is a sexually transmitted disease which presents in stages:

**Primary stage:** It is characterized by the appearance of a **painless** papule on penis 1-3 weeks after sexual contact. It may ulcerate or go unnoticed.

Extragenital presentation is on fingers or tongue.

**Secondary stage:** It appears 2-6 weeks later. The patient presents with painful regional lymphadenopathy in the groin—the enlarged lymph nodes are called **buboes.**

**Tertiary stage:** It is seen in untreated patients. It is characterized by fibrosis and scarring, which can lead to urethral or rectal strictures.

**Non-gonococcal urethritis:** Chlamydia is one of the **common** causes of NGU (30%). Other organisms include—*Ureaplasma urealyticum, Mycoplasma genitalium, Mycoplasma hominis, C. trachomatis, Herpesvirus, Cytomegalovirus* and *Trichomonas vaginalis.*

## C. pneumoniae

It causes lower respiratory tract infections that evolve into bronchopneumonia. TW-183 and AR-39, originally known as **TWAR strains** are now known as *C. pneumoniae.*

## C. psittaci

It is the only zoonotic *Chlamydia* species pathogenic for humans. Birds particularly parrot and parakeets and pigeons are its normal hosts. The disease is **psittacosis (or ornithosis).**

The disease is systemic and lungs are primarily infected. It causes influenza like syndrome—headache, fever, malaise, cough and anorexia.

## Epidemiology

***C. trachomatis*** is a strict human pathogen with person to person transmission.

***C. psittaci*** is transmitted to man by inhalation of air-borne particles (usually dried bird droppings).

***C. pneumoniae*** is a strict human pathogen with a person to person transmission.

## Laboratory Diagnosis

The samples for diagnosis of chlamydial infections are collected as mucosal scrapings. **Endocervical swab** in female and **urethral** samples in males are the best samples.

Since, *Chlamydia* are intracellular organisms, they **cannot be cultured** on bacteriological media. However, they can be **grown on cell culture** monolayers.

Although there are many antigenic detection methods for *C. trachomatis,* culture remains the most sensitive and specific method of detection of all *Chlamydia* species.

### Direct Detection

**Antigenic detection**

- Immunofluorescence using radiolabelled monoclonal antibodies against species-specific MOMP or genus specific LPS.
- Enzyme immunoassay.
- Nucleic acid hybridization using DNA probes and PCR for gene amplification.

**Chlamydial culture in cell monolayers**

Growth in McCoy cell lines (irradiated mouse fibroblast cells), HeLa cells, BHK-21 (baby hamster kidney) can be done.

*Detection is by:*

- Iodine staining for inclusion bodies.
- Giemsa staining.
- Fluorescent labelled monoclonal antibodies.
- Immunofluorescence.

## Serology

It is done for IgG or IgM antibody detection. The methods used are ELISA and immunofluorescence. A specific IgM ELISA is done for detection of neonatal pneumonia.

## Treatment

**Tetracycline** is the drug of choice for trachoma and inclusion conjunctivitis. In younger children, erythromycin is given.

Oral and topical erythromycin is administered in ophthalmia neonatorum.

Tetracycline is used for genital infections by *C. trachomatis* and also for psittacosis and pneumonia due to *C. pneumoniae.*

In LGV, Tetracycline and sulphonamides are given for 3 weeks

Summary of Rickettsial, Ehrlichial and Bartonella diseases

| *Disease* | | *Organism* | *Arthropod Vector* | *Mammalian Reservoir* |
|---|---|---|---|---|
| Typhus group | Epidemic typhus Brill Zinsser disease | *Rickettsia prowazekii* | Louse | Humans |
| | Endemic typhus | *Rickettsia typhi* | Flea | Rodents |
| | Scrub typhus | *Rickettsia (Orientia) tsutsugamushi* | Mite | Rodents |
| Spotted fevers | Rocky Mountain Spotted Fever | *Rickettsia rickettsia* | Tick | Rodents, dogs |
| | Rickettsial pox | *Rickettsia akari* | Mite | Mice |
| | Mediterranean spotted fever, Indian tick typhus | *Rickettsia conorii* | Tick | Rodents, dogs |
| Q fever | Q fever | *Coxiella burnetii* | Airborne, fomites, no vector for human disease | Sheep, cattle goat |
| Ehrlichiae | Human monocyte ehrlichiosis | *Ehrlichia chaffeensis* | Tick | Deer |
| | Human monocyte | *Neorickettsia* | Trematode infected | Unknown |

*Contd.*

*Contd.*

| | | | | |
|---|---|---|---|---|
| | ehrlichiosis | *sennetsu* | fish? | |
| | Human granulocyte ehrlichiosis | *Anaplasma phago cytophilum* | Tick | Mice |
| | Human granulocyte ehrlichiosis | *Ehrlichia ewingii* | Tick | Dogs |
| Barto-nellae | Bacillary angiomato-sis, Oroya fever, Carrion's disease | *Bartonella bacillifor-mis* | | |
| | Cat scratch disease | *Bartonella henselae* | | |
| | Trench fever | *Bartonella quintana* (formerly *Rochalimea quintana)* | Louse | Humans |

## CHAPTER THREE

# Immunology

### BASIC CONCEPTS OF IMMUNITY

**Immunity** refers to body's ability to resist any type of foreign substances like microbes or toxins, which are potentially damaging to the body.

Some microbes, such as viruses, infect individual cells; others, including many bacteria, divide extra-cellularly within tissues or the body cavities. Human body has evolved to protect us from diverse pathogens using different components of the immune system.

### Components of Immune System

- Cells
- Soluble mediators

### Cells of Immune System

Originate in bone marrow, migrate to patrol the tissues, circulating in the blood and in a specialized system of vessels called the lymphatic system.

The cells, which mediate immunity mainly include lymphocytes and phagocytes.

**Lymphocytes** that form a part of adaptive immune system, recognize antigens on pathogens. They have specialized functions.

- **B cells** (mature in bone marrow) which when activated differentiate into **plasma cells** that make antibodies. B cells usually recognize intact antigen molecules.
- **T cells** (mature in thymus) have two main classes.
- One includes **cytotoxic T cells-Tc** [recognized by surface marker **CD8** (cluster designation)].

- other includes **helper T cells-TH2** and **inflammatory T cells-TH1** [recognized by surface marker **CD4**] coordinate the immune response by direct cell-cell interactions and the release of cytokines that help B cells to make antibodies.

T lymphocytes recognize antigen fragments on the surface of other cells of the body.

Lymphocytes continually recirculate from bloodstream through peripheral lymphoid organs like spleen, lymph nodes and mucosa/gut associated lymphoid tissue.

**Phagocytes**, which form a part of innate immune system internalize or engulf pathogens and degrade them. Two main phagocytes are:

- **Macrophages:** Also act as antigen presenting cells, secrete inflammatory cytokines and thus form a part of innate as well as adaptive immune response.
- **Neutrophils** (polymorphonuclear cells or PMNs): Main cell type in initial phases of inflammatory response, do not present antigens, so are part of innate system only.

*Other cells include:*

- **Eosinophils**: Important chiefly in defense against parasitic infections
- **Basophils**: Release histamine in allergic responses
- **NK cells** (natural killer): Large lymphocytes that nonspecifically destroy foreign cells, tumour cells and virus infected **cells**
- **LAK cells** (lymphokine activated killer): Activated cells that play role in antibody dependent cell mediated cytotoxicity (ADCC).

### Soluble Mediators of Immunity

- **Immunoglobulins**: Surface molecules on B cells secreted as antibodies in response to antigenic stimulation
- **Cytokines**: Chemical mediators involved in signaling between cells during immune response.

- **Complement**: Group of proteins which interact sequentially on activation and result in lysis or opsonization of bacteria and chemotaxis of phagocytes.

## Types of Immunity

**Exterior defenses**: **First line of defense** is the intact skin and mucous membranes.

**Innate (nonadaptive) immunity**: If microorganisms breach external defenses and enter the body, then the innate arm of the immune system **(Second line of defense)** comes into action. Components of innate system are preformed and fully active, so can act immediately. The action of innate components is non-specific. Innate immune responses play a crucial part in initiation and subsequent direction of adaptive immune responses. Moreover, since there is a delay of four to five days before initial adaptive immune response takes effect, innate response has a critical role in controlling infections during this period.

**Adaptive (acquired) immunity**: Important difference between these is that an adaptive immune response (Third line of defense) is highly specific for a particular pathogen and can respond to millions of different antigens. Moreover, adaptive responses improve with the successive encounter with the same pathogen (**secondary response** is much more vigorous than the **primary response**). In effect, adaptive immune system 'remembers' the infectious agent (**immunological memory**). Thus key features of adaptive immune response are **diversity**, **specificity** and **memory**.

## Cellular and Humoral Immunity

Adaptive immunity has two components

- **Humoral immunity** mediated by immunoglobulins is a major defense to opsonize most bacterial infections and neutralize toxins.

- **Cellular immunity** mediated by T lymphocytes is mainly responsible for defense against tumor cells and infections due to viruses, fungi, parasites and certain intracellular bacteria like *Mycobacterium tuberculosis*.

### Active and Passive Immunity

- **Active immunity** is generated by the body's own immune system; **long lasting, slow onset.**
  *Natural active immunity*—produced by exposure to infection.
  *Acquired active immunity*—produced by exposure to vaccines.
- **Passive immunity** is not generated by the body's own immune system, preformed in another host; **prompt availability, short lifespan**.
  *Natural passive immunity*—antibodies transferred transplacentally from mother to the newborn.
  *Acquired passive immunity*—injecting immunoglobulins for treating diseases.

### Immunological Tolerance

Human immune system can differentiate foreign or non-self-antigens from self. This self-tolerance prevents the body from mounting an immune response against its own tissues. This tolerance is acquired during embryonic development of the immune system. This is carried out by a combination of **negative and positive selection** of lymphocytes. This results in deletion of differentiating T and B cells specific against autoantigens.

Immune system may breakdown leading to immunodeficiency or hypersensitivity or autoimmune diseases.

## MECHANISM OF IMMUNE RESPONSE

**Antigen** (***gen***erate ***anti***bodies)

Usually a high molecular weight protein, but may also be a low molecular weight protein or a high molecular weight polysaccharide (e.g. dextran).

The specificity of an antigen is due to specific areas of its molecules called **determinant sites** or **epitopes.** One protein has several epitopes and these may differ from each other not only in their specificity but also in their antigenic potency.

### Hapten

A hapten is usually a non-protein substance which has little or no antigenic property by itself but which combines with a protein to form a new antigen which is capable of stimulating production of specific immunoglobulins, the specificity of which depends upon the hapten fraction rather than the carrier protein.

A secondary response can be obtained by subsequent challenge by the same carrier hapten complex but not by the hapten combined with a different carrier. The haptens, however, do not require the protein carrier to react with the antibody produced.

Lipids and simple carbohydrates which are not antigenic and the more complex polysaccharides which are poorly antigenic produce powerful antigens when they are combined with protein.

### Adjuvant

Immunogenicity of an antigen can be improved by combining it with some protein molecules called adjuvants. Example, in DPT vaccine pertussis component acts as an adjuvant to diphtheria and tetanus toxoids.

### Recognition of Antigens

**Antigen receptors on lymphocytes**: T lymphocytes have antigen specific receptors. In B lymphocytes, immunoglobulins present on cell surface serve as receptors for antigens.

**Antigen processing and presentation:** Pathogens or their toxic products in the extracellular spaces of the body are bound by immunoglobulins secreted as antibodies by activated B cells. Binding by antibody neutralizes viruses, and marks pathogens for destruction by phagocytes and complement.

Intracellular pathogens and their products can be found in two compartments—either the **cytoplasmic or vesicular compartment** of the cells.

T cells can detect cells infected with intracellular pathogens because such cells display on their surface protein fragments derived from pathogen's proteins. These foreign peptides are delivered to the cell surface by specialized cellular proteins called the **major histocompatibility complex (MHC) molecules**. Just as specific blood groups are responsible for transfusion reactions, likewise specific MHC molecules are responsible for graft rejection following tissue or organ transplantation. In man the MHC antigens are referred to as **Human leucocyte antigens (HLA)** and are coded by genes located on the short arm of chromosome 6.

Two types of MHC molecules:

- **Class I**—present on all nucleated cells
- **Class II**—present on antigen presenting cells.

MHC class I molecules present antigens from pathogens in cytosol to CD8 cytotoxic T cells, which once activated generally kill any cell they specifically recognize. Therefore, this type of immune response is important in countering intracellular organisms for example viruses or some bacteria and fungi. Non-nucleated cells like RBCs do not express MHC class I, therefore malarial parasite can live in this privileged site.

MHC II molecules are normally found on B cells, dendritic cells and macrophages—cells that participate in immune responses—but not on other tissue cells. When helper CD4 cells (TH2) recognize antigen bound to MHC class II molecules on B cells, they stimulate the B cells to produce antibodies. Likewise, inflammatory CD4 T cells (TH1) recognize antigens bound to MHC class II molecules on macrophages. This leads to activation of these cells to destroy the pathogens in their vesicles.

MHC molecules are **polygenic**—several genes code for them and polymorphic—there are multiple alleles of each gene. Any T cell can recognize antigen only when presented with a particular set of MHC molecules. This is called **MHC restriction**.

HLA typing is important in organ transplantation.

## IMMUNOGLOBULINS, CYTOKINES AND COMPLEMENT

### Immunoglobulins

The immunoglobulin molecules on the plasma membrane of B—lymphocytes are integral membrane proteins. Free immunoglobulins function as antibodies.

#### *Structure of Immunoglobulins*

An immunoglobulin molecule is made of 2 heavy and 2 light chains. Disulphide bonds anchor the light chain and also hold the two heavy chains together. The heavy chains are of two subtypes: μ, γ, α, ε, δ (constituting respectively IgM, IgG, IgA, IgE and IgD). The light chains are of two types: **kappa and lambda**. The $NH_2$ terminal half of each chain ( designated as $V_L$ in the light chain and $V_H$ in the heavy chain), has a variable sequence of amino acids and is, therefore, called the **'variable region'**. The COOH terminal half has a relatively constant sequence and is called the **'constant region'**.

Disulphide bonds fold each chain into incomplete loops. There are 4 loops in the heavy chain of which only one (designated as VH) lies in the variable region and the 3 others (designated as CH1, CH2 and CH3) lie in the constant region. Each light chain, however, has only two loops, 1 in the variable region (designated as VL) and one in the constant region (designated as CL). The variable region bind to the antigen. The CH2 in IgG binds to complement C1q.

The immunoglobulin molecule can also be split enzymatically by papain or pepsin.

- Papain yeilds Fab (antigen binding fraction) which bears all the 'variable regions' and Fc (crystallisable fraction). Fc determines such properties of the immunoglobulin as diffusibility, placental transfer, complement fixation, opsonization, etc.
- Pepsin yields a dimer of Fab (designated as F(ab)2) and the COOH halves of the heavy chains.

## Types of Immunoglobulins

### *IgM*

- IgM comprise about 10% of the total plasma immunoglobulins.
- It is the predominant immunoglobulin produced in the primary response. It appears early in the secondary response but its level does not rise significantly thereafter.
- Also because of its large size, it is predominantly intravascular. This, coupled with its early production makes it important in bacteremias.
- IgM is the only immunoglobulin which is **produced before birth.** Natural antibodies like anti-A and anti-B are therefore if the IgM type.
- It has a theoretical valency of 10 which is actually observed in cases of small haptens. With larger ones, its effective valency drops to 5, perhaps due to stearic restriction due to lack of flexibility in the molecule. However, it has much more affinity and avidity of binding for large antigens with multiple epitopes than for small haptens.
- IgM causes **very effective agglutination.** It produces **complement fixation** by the classical pathway and the lysis It causes thereby is very effective. Its opsonizing power is however rather weak.

### *IgG*

- IgG is the **most abundant immunoglobulin** comprising about 70% of the total immunoglobulins.

- It is the major immunoglobulin to be synthesized during the **secondary response** in which the initial IgM production gives way to IgG production (**class switch**).
- Unlike IgM, it is **able to cross the placenta.** Thus it is able to provide passive immunity to the neonate in its first few weeks. The protection is further reinforced by the transfer of colostral IgG across the gut mucosa of the neonates. After birth, the serum IgG concentration steadily falls for 2-3 months and then rises slowly over years.
- IgG readily **diffuses out into the extravascular spaces** where its concentration is the same as that in the plasma. It is also found in the milk, saliva, nasal and bronchial secretions.
- IgG causes opsonisation, ADCC and neutralisation of toxins. Although it fixes complement by the classical pathway, the lysis it produces through complement fixation is weak. The IgG antigen complex binds to platelet through Fc receptors causing **platelet aggregation.**

*IgA*

- The intestinal mucosa secretes IgA bound to a secretory protein which stabilises it against proteolysis.
- It **coats the microbes and inhibits their adherence to the mucosal cells** thereby preventing the entry into the body tissues. *Neisseria gonorrhoea* which produces IgA protease can penetrate the mucosal barrier even in the immune person.
- IgA appears in colostrum, saliva, nasal and lung secretions, tears, genitourinary and gastrointestinal fluids. IgA effects **opsonisation and neutralisation.** It also fixes the complement by the alternate pathway.

*IgE*

- The antigen-IgE complex binds to mast cells and basophils.

- This causes degranulation of the mast cells with the release of anaphylatoxins (SRS A), mast cell chemotactic factor, eosinophil chemotactic factor, etc.
- Haptens with a single epitope which cannot cross-link Fc receptors cannot degranulate mast cells; in fact, they inhibit it by blocking the Fab of the IgE. Parasites are particularly efficient in stimulating IgE production.

*IgD*

- They are present on the surface of the B cells and are known to act as antigen receptors for the B cells. However, their significance is not understood.

*Cytokines*

Cytokines can be best defined as small proteins that usually act in an autocrine (on the cell that produced them) or paracrine (on cells close by) manner. Some common cytokines are :

**Interleukins**: IL1, IL2, IL4, IL10, IL12.

- IL1—secreted by macrophages, activate lymphocytes.
- IL2—secreted by T cells, cause T cell proliferation and differentiation.
- IL4, IL5—secreted by B cells, cause B cell growth and differentiation.
- IL10—secreted by T cells, inhibits TH1 response.
- IL12—secreted by monocytes, induce TH1 response.

**Interferons**: IFNα, IFNβ, IFNγ.

- IFNα—secreted by B cells, MHC class I induction, antiviral state and NK cell stimulation.
- IFNβ—secreted by fibroblasts, MHC class I induction, antiviral and antiproliferative.
- IFNγ—secreted by T cells, MHC class I and II induction, macrophage activation, antiviral and antiproliferative.

**Tumour necrosis factor**—TNFα, TNFβ.

Growth Factors

**Colony stimulating factors**—G-CSF, GM-CSF.

**Chemokines**: Migration inhibition factor, macrophage chemotactic factor, etc.

## Complement System

The complement system is a system of 9 enzymatic proteins designated C1 to C9 present in the blood as plasma proteins. Normally in the inactive state, their activity is triggered when C1 binds to the antigen-antibody complex.

The activated C1 in turn activates the other complements in a series of cascade reactions. While the final product of complement activation is a **membrane attack complex (MAC)** which is cytolytic, the other by products cause vasodilatation, chemotaxis, immune adherence and mast cell degranulation.

The antibodies, which can thus 'fix' and thereby activate the complement pathway, are IgM and IgG. IgA also fixes the complement but does so by the "**alternate pathway**" and not by the "**classical pathway**" as in the case of IgM.

### *Lectin Pathway*

There is another pathway of complement activation that intersects the classical pathway but is activated in an antibody-independent fusion. The activation is initiated by mannan binding lectin (MBL), which bind to two serine proteinases to lead to antibody independent activation of the classical pathway.

## Clinical Implications and Future Perspectives

In normal course of infection, adaptive immune response clears the infection and establishes a state of protective immunity. However, derangement or failure of the immune response can lead to various disease conditions.

- **Immunodeficiency diseases**

Conditions where the defense mechanism of the body is impaired leading to repeated microbial infections. These infections can even be caused by the organisms **(opportunistic infections)** which normally are resisted by the healthy bodies.

Immunodeficiency can occur in: B cells, T cells, complement or phagocytes

> Recurrent infections with pyogenic bacteria like staphylococci indicate **B cell deficiency**, whereas recurrent infections with viruses, fungi or protozoa indicate **T cell deficiency**

Immunodeficiency diseases can be classified into:

- **Primary/Congenital:** Those in which genetic errors can lead to impairment of any component of the immune system like humoral or cellular.
- **Secondary/Acquired:** Following conditions that lead to impairment of the immune response; as malnutrition, drugs, radiation or infections like HIV.

> **Congenital immunodeficiencies**:
>
> **B cell deficiencies**
>
> - **X-linked hypogammaglobulinemia (Bruton's agammaglobulinemia)**: Absence of B cells, very low immunoglobulin levels; common in boys; mutant tyrosine kinase; recurrent bacterial infections.
> - **Selective immunoglobulin deficiencies**: IgA deficiency most common; recurrent lung and sinus infections.
>
> **T cell deficiencies**
>
> - **Thymic aplasia (DiGeorge's syndrome)**: Absence of T cells; defective development of pharyngeal pouches; not a genetic disease.
> - **Chronic mucocutaneous candidiasis**: Deficient T cell response specifically against *Candida.*
>
> **Combined B Cell and T Cell deficiencies**
>
> - **Severe combined immunodeficiency syndrome**: Deficiency of both B and T cells; defective IL-2

receptor, absence of MHC II proteins, ADA or PNP deficiency; may have bare lymphocyte syndrome.

- **Wiskott-Aldrich syndrome**: X-linked disease, seen only in males; inability to mount IgM response to bacterial capsular polysaccharide

**Complement deficiencies**

- **Hereditary angioedema**: Deficiency of C1 protease inhibitor; too much C3a, C5a; laryngeal edema

**Phagocyte deficiencies**

**Complement deficiencies**

- **Chronic granulomatous disease**: No oxidative burst; lack of NADPH oxidase; diagnosed by nitroblue tetrazolium dye reduction test or DCF test.
- **Chediak Higashi syndrome**: Autosomal recessive disease; failure of formation of phagolysosomes of neutrophils.
- **Job's syndrome (Hyper IgE syndrome)**: recurrent 'cold'; failure to produce gamma interferon

**Acquired immunodeficiency syndrome (AIDS)**, a disease that is currently a major worldwide problem, is unique in that **HIV (human immunodeficiency virus),** the retrovirus that causes many cases of it, binds to CD4 and produces a decrease in the number of CD4 helper T cells. The loss of helper lymphocytes leads in turn to failure of proliferation of CD8 and B cells, with eventual loss of immune function and death from infections due to normally non-pathogenic bacteria or cancer.

- **Hypersensitivity**

When an immune response results in considerable damage to the body, it is called hypersensitivity. There are mainly four types of hypersensitivity reactions:

**Type I (Anaphylaxis):** This occurs due to mast cell degranulation and is caused by antigens which evoke a strong IgE response. Allergic asthma and food allergies are examples of such reactions.

**Type II (Antibody-mediated cytotoxicity):** It involves combination of immunoglobulins (IgG and IgM) with foreign antigenic components on a cell surface leading to its degradation. Example of this is seen in haemolytic disease of the newborn. The antibodies react with the antigens on the RBCs of the newborn and irreversibly destroy them.

**Type III (Immune complex disorders):** The antigen antibody complex is deposited in various normal tissues of the body where it fixes the complement. Complement activation damages the tissue cells in the vicinity. A form of glomerulonephritis (damage to the glomeruli of the kidney) is an example of this form.

**Type IV (Delayed type hypersensitivity):** It is the outcome of cell-mediated immunity in tissues of sensitized individuals. Sensitized T lymphocytes and macrophages mediate the damage here. Classical example is seen in tuberculosis.

**Type V (Simulating antibody** type): Seen in Graves' disease.

- **Autoimmunity**

Normally human body does not evoke immune response against its own tissue. However, sometimes antibodies or T cells may be formed against own tissue leading to autoimmune diseases. Examples include **myasthenia gravis** (autoantibodies against motor end plate), **pernicious anaemia** (autoantibodies against gastric mucosa) and **Hashimoto's disease** (autoantibodies against the thyroid).

The possible mechanisms of development of autoimmunity could be:

- Clones of cells with immunological reactivity with self-antigens called **forbidden clones** are eliminated in embryonic life. Their persistence or development in later life by somatic mutation can lead to autoimmunity.

- A sequestered 'self' antigen which did not come in contact with, and thereby deplete its corresponding clone during foetal life will elicit an immune response in the adult if it came in contact with immunocompetent cells.
- Although antibodies are highly specific, in some cases, an antibody formed in response to some foreign antigen cross-reacts with some tissue of the body itself. This is certainly the case in rheumatic heart disease where the heart is damaged by antibodies formed against streptococcal infections.
- With age or exposure to chemical agents, some tissues of the body may undergo an antigenic variation, which is not recognized as 'self'. $T_s$ cells (suppressor cells, a subpopulation of T cells) may fail to check the immune process adequately

Important autoimmune diseases

| *Autoimmune disease* | *Target of immune response* |
|---|---|
| Myasthenia gravis | Acetylcholine receptor |
| Graves' disease | TSH receptor |
| SLE | dsDNA, histones |
| Rheumatoid arthritis | IgG in joints |
| Rheumatic fever | Heart and joint tissue |
| ITP | Platelet membrane |
| Goodpasture's syndrome | Basement membrane of kidney, lungs |
| Hashimoto's thyroiditis | Thyroglobulin |
| Gullian-Barré syndrome | Myelin protein |
| Multiple sclerosis | Reaction to myelin protein causes demyelination of brain neurons |

Microbes associated with autoimmune diseases

| *Organism* | *Disease* |
|---|---|
| *Streptococcus pyogenes* | Rheumatic fever |
| *Campyloacter jejuni* | Gullian Barré syndrome |
| *Echerichia coli* | Primary biliary cirrhosis |
| *Chlamydia trachomatis* | Reiter's syndrome |
| *Yersinia enterocolitica* | Graves' disease |
| Hepatitis B virus | Multiple sclerosis |
| Hepatitis C virus | Mixed cryoglobulinemia |

## Tolerance to Foetus

Because of the incorporation of the paternal genes, the foetus differs in genetic make up from its mother. It should therefore induce immune response in the mother in much the same way as does the foetal Rhesus antigen in an Rh mother. That, however, never happens. The reason could be as follows:

- The placenta is shielded from immunological attack because after implantation, the cells of the trophoblasts lose much of their immunogenicity due to:
  - A decrease in the density of the MHC antigens
  - Development of an inert coating mucoprotein on the surface of these cells.
- **Alpha-fetoprotein** (AFP) produced during embryonic development is a generalised immunosuppressive. So may be progesterone.
- The **anti-MHC antibodies** produced by the mother are specifically absorbed by the placenta and denied entry into foetal circulation.
- It is suggested that when the foetus encounters maternal T cells at the placenta, the foetal T cells are activated and suppress the mother's T cells.

## Tissue/Organ Transplant

Transplantation has become possible because of extensive knowledge about manipulation and controlling the immune response. Tissue or organ transplanted from donor to recipient is known as the graft. Only those grafts in which there is a complete identity between the genetic constitution of the donor and recipient survive and function. Therefore, blood grouping and HLA matching is essential to prevent graft rejection. Hence best chances of graft survival is amongst identical twins.

A number of treatments have been developed to overcome the rejection of transplanted organs in humans. The goal of treatment is to stop rejection without leaving the patient vulnerable to massive infections. One approach is to kill T lymphocytes by killing all rapidly dividing cells with drugs such as azathioprine, a purine antimetabolite. Another is to administer glucocorticoids or immunomodulators as cyclosporine and rapamycin.

**Autograft**: Transfer of an individual's own tissue to another site of the body
**Syngenic graft** (isograft): Transfer of tissue between genetically identical individuals, e.g. identical twins
**Xenograft** (heterograft): Transfer of tissue between different species
**Allograft** (homograft): Graft between genetically different members of the same species, e.g. one human to another
**Allograft rejection**: Acceptance or rejection determined, in large part, by class I and class II MHC proteins on donor cells. Major role is played by **Class II**, especially **DR** locus coded proteins.
**Acute reaction**:
- **Primary (first-set reaction)**: T-cell mediated reaction is the main cause of reaction; 11-14 days; **CD-8 cytotoxic T** cells do most of the killing of allograft cells
- **Accelerated (second-set reaction)**: If a second allograft from the same donor is applied to a sensitized recipient, it is rejected in 5-6 days.

**Chronic rejection:** Months to years after transplantation; main pathologic finding is atherosclerosis of vascular endothelium; immunologic basis unclear; incompatibility of minor histocompatibility antigens and side effect of immunosuppressive drugs likely reasons.
**Hyperacute rejection:** Typically within minutes of transplantation; due to reaction of preformed anti ABO antibodies; also called '**white graft**', therefore ABO blood group matching and crossmatching is a must.
**Graft- versus-Host reaction**: This reaction occurs as a result of presence of immunocompetent T cells from the donor in the graft, which destroy recipient's cells considering them foreign. Also occurs following blood transfusion in an immunocompromised individual.

### Immunotherapy

This is being increasingly perceived as the future of modern therapy. Active and passive immunizations are in fact forms of immunotherapy. It can be used not only in preventing or treating infectious diseases but also in limiting tumors.

### Vaccination

It is a form of active acquired immunity. The principle use of a vaccine is to use the host immune response to prevent disease.

The various types are:

- **Killed**: Use purified and inactivated organisms, e.g. pertussis, rabies and hepatitis A vaccines
- **Live attenuated**: Utilize mutants that are antigenically related to the wild strains but do not cause disease, e.g. oral polio and mumps vaccine.
- **Synthetic peptide**: Antigenically active polypeptides are synthesized and used as vaccines, e.g. hepatitis B and influenza vaccines.
- **Subunit vaccines**: Only those components of the organisms that evoke a protective immune response are used as vaccine, e.g. cholera vaccine.
- **DNA vaccines**: Gene guns are used to deliver naked DNA into the host, where it is taken up by the cells to produce protective antibodies. It is a potential candidate as HIV vaccine.

### Monoclonal Antibodies (MoAb)

These are antibodies against a single epitope of an antigen, i.e. high specificity. Large quantities of monoclonal antibodies can be produced by fusing a single plasma cell or spleen cell with a tumour cell (**hybridoma** technique). Newer technique of producing monoclonal antibodies involves fusion of antibody producing genes with bacteriophages (virus infecting bacteria). When they infect a bacteria, required antibodies are expressed and can be purified (**phage display technique**).

MoAb can be used in:

- **Diagnosis**: Used in *in vitro* antigen antibody reaction like precipitation, agglutination and neutralisation reactions.
- **Treatment**: Used as immunotherapy for infectious and non-infectious diseases.
- **Research**: Discovery of new pathogens and their mechanism of causing disease.

CHAPTER FOUR

# Medical Mycology

Fungi are eukaryotic. Although many fungi are medically important as pathogens and cause spoilage of fruits, grains or vegetables, they are also used in production of foods (e.g. breads, cheese, wine, beer) and antibiotics.

Two medically important fungal structures:

- **Chitin** (composed of N-acetylglucosamine): Present in fungal cell wall (unlike peptidoglycans in bacteria), makes fungi insensitive to antibiotics like penicillins.
- **Ergosterol:** Present in fungal cell membrane (unlike cholesterol in human cell membrane). Antifungal drugs like Amphotericin B and fluconazole or ketoconazole have selective action against fungal cell membrane.

Two forms of fungi:

- **Yeast:** Single celled, reproduce by budding.
- **Molds:** Long filaments (hyphae) and form mycelium.

Some fungi show **thermal dimorphism**, i.e. exist as hyphae at room temperature (25°C) and as yeasts at body temperature (37°C). These are called dimorphic fungi.

### Fungi Reproduce Either:

- Sexually forming **sexual spores (ascospore, basidiospore and zygospore)**. Fungi are classified on the basis of sexual spores. Ascospores are formed in a sac called ascus, basidiospores are formed externally on the tip of a pedestal, zygospores are single large spores with thick walls)

- Asexually forming **asexual spores (conidia)**. Most fungi multiply asexually. The shape, size, number and distribution of asexual spores helps in identification and differentiation of fungi. Examples of asexual spores:
  - **Arthrospores**: *Coccidioides immitis*
  - **Chlamydospores**: *Candida albicans*
  - **Blastospores** (budding): yeasts
  - **Sporangiospores**: *Mucor, Rhizopus*
  - Micro and macro **aleurispores**: dermatophytes.

Sexual form of fungi is known as teleomorph; asexual form is known as anamorph.
**Anamorph + Telemorph = Holomorph**
e.g. Holomorph of Cryptococcus would be : *Filobasidiella (Cryptococcus) neoformans*
Classification of fungi is based on their teleomorph

**Fungal spores** are sexual or asexual, for reproduction; one fungus can produce many spores
**Bacterial spores** are for survival, not reproduction; one bacterium can produce one spore

**Laboratory diagnosis** of fungal diseases:

- **Direct microscopic examination**:
  - **10% KOH** dissolves tissue and keratin, and fungi can be seen better especially for skin, hair nail infections, e.g. dermatophytes
  - **India ink** preparation of spinal fluid for *Cryptococcus neoformans*
  - **Calcofluor white** is fluorescent and used for tissue specimens
  - **Methenamine-silver stain** for diagnosis of fungi in tissue.
- **Culture**
  - Sabouraud's dextrose agar **(SDA)** with or without chloramphenicol and cyclohexamide; incubated at 25°C

- Brain heart infusion agar (**BHIA**) used to demonstrate dimorphism (yeast forms seen at 37°C in dimorphic fungi)
- Growth stained with lactophenol cotton blue (**LPCB**) and watched microscopically. Lactic acid acts as hydrant, phenol as disinfectant and cotton blue is the dye
- Molds are differentiated on the basis of **morphological differences** (septate/ aseptate hyphae, branching, type/ number/ arrangement/ distribution of spores, specialized structures)
- Yeast may have to be distinguished on the basis of **assimilation reactions** (anabolic reactions unlike bacterial biochemical differentiation which are catabolic reactions).

- **DNA probe tests**
  - Available for *Coccidioides, Histoplasma, Blastomyces, Cryptococcus*
  - Help in early diagnosis in culture.
- **Serologic tests**
  - Used mainly for systemic mycosis
  - Significant rise in antibody titer is required to confirm diagnosis
  - **Complement fixation** most frequently used for coccidioidomycosis, histoplasmosis, blastomycosis
  - **Latex agglutination test** done for detection of polysaccharide capsular antigen in cryptococcosis.

Medically important fungi belong mainly to three phyla based on sexual spores:

*Ascomycota*: Most medically important fungi belong to this group, e.g.:

- Cutaneous fungi: Dermatophytes
- Subcutaneous dimorphic fungi: *Sporothrix schenkii*
- Systemic dimorphic fungi: *Histoplasma, Coccidioides*
- Yeast like fungi: *Candida*

> - Dematiaceous fungi (Black molds): *Fonsecaea, Phialophora, Cladosporium*
> - Laboratory contaminants: *Curvalaria, Alternaria, Aspergillus*
>
> ***Basidiomycota***: *Cryptococcus, Malasezzia furfur*, Mushrooms
>
> ***Zygomycota***: *Mucor, Rhizopus, Absidia, Cunninghamella, Saxenaceae*

Medical mycoses can be divided into four categories:

- **Cutaneous**
- **Subcutaneous**
- **Systemic**
- **Opportunistic.**

## CUTANEOUS MYCOSES

### Dermatophytoses (Tinea, Ringworm)

- Caused by dermatophytes that infect only superficial keratinized structures (skin, hair and nails), and are spread by direct contact.

Three important genera:

- ***Trichophyton***—infects hair, nail and skin
- ***Microsporum*** (also spread by animals)—infects hair and skin
- ***Epidermophyton***—infects nail and skin.

These are chronic infections located in warm humid areas of the body.

| | |
|---|---|
| Tinea capitis: scalp | Tinea pedis: foot (athlete's foot) |
| Tinea cruris: groin (jock itch) | Tinea barbae: beard region |
| Tinea corporis: body/trunk | Tinea unguium: nails |
| Tinea favosa: favus (honeycomb) caused by *Trichophyton schoenleinii* | |
| Tinea manuum: palmar area of hands | |

- *T. tonsurans, T. violaceum* and *T. schoenleinii* cause **endothrix**
- *T. rubrum* and *T mentagrophytes* form **red pigment**, differentiated by **hair perforation test**
- *Microsporum* species show **fluorescence** when exposed to UV light in **Wood's lamp. Splendore-Hoeppli phenomenon** (eosinophilic infiltrates around lesions) may be seen in tissue
- Treatment involves local antifungal creams (miconazole, tolnaftate, undecylenic acid) or oral griseofulvin.
- **"Id" (dermatophytid) reaction** is a hypersensitivity response in one skin location (e.g., fingers, to the presence of the organisms in another e.g., feet.

### Tinea (Pityriasis) Versicolor

- Caused by *Malassezia furfur (*member of Phylum *Basidiomycota)*, only cosmetic significance. Characterized by hypopigmented areas, especially on tanned skin, slight scaling or itching.
- On KOH preparation, **tissue dimorphism** seen, typical **"grapes and bananas"** or **"spaghetti and meatball"** appearance. Culture can be done on SDA with **olive oil** overlay.
- Topical miconazole is treatment of choice

**Tinea nigra**—caused by *Hortae (Exophiala) werneckii*

**White piedra**—caused by *Trichosporon* species

**Black piedra**—caused by *Piedraria hortae.*

## SUBCUTANEOUS MYCOSES

Generally caused by fungi in soil and enter body through trauma.

### Sporotrichosis

- Caused by *Sporothrix schenckii*, a dimorphic fungus.

- Typically results from a **thorn injury** e.g., gardeners who prune roses or while handling plants, moss and wood.
- Local abscess or ulcer with nodules in draining lymphatics.
- Round or **cigar-shaped** budding yeasts seen in tissue specimens.
- In culture, **daisy head** appearance due to flower like distribution of conidia.
- Drug of choice is itraconazole.

### Mycetoma

- Soil organisms enter through wounds and cause swelling and abscesses with pus containing granules discharging through the sinuses.
- Fungal mycetomas are called **Eumycotic mycetomas**, caused by *Madurella madurai* (madura foot), *Petriellidium*, etc.
- Actinomycetes like *Nocardia* can cause **actinomycotic mycetomas**. Splendore—Hoeppli phenomenon is seen (e.g. with *Actinomyces israelli*)
- Differentiation done by KOH examination and Gram staining.
- Bacterial mycetomas treated by sulfonamides while in fungal, surgical excision is recommended as effective drugs are not available yet.

### Chromoblastomycosis (Chromomycosis)

- Slowly progressive granulomatous infection caused by several **dematiaceous** fungi (Black molds) from soil.
- Term black molds is now replaced by **"Phaeoid"** hyphae.
- These fungi (*Fonseceae, Phialophora, Cladosporium*, etc.) produce melanin like pigment.
- Characterized by presence of **'muriform cells'** or **'sclerotic bodies'**.
- Infections causes by black molds are collectively known as **"Phaeohyphomycosis"** (if muriform cells are not seen) while infections caused by fungi

having hyaline hyphae are called **"Hyalohyphomycosis"**.

- Treated with oral flucytosine or thiabendazole, plus local surgery.

## SYSTEMIC MYCOSES

Invariably result from inhalation of spores of dimorphic fungi that have mold forms in the soil. Within the lungs, the spores differentiate into yeasts or other specialized structures.

### *Coccidioides*

- *Coccidioides immitis* causes coccidioidomycosis, infection of the lungs.
- Dimorphic fungus that forms mold (hyphae with alternating **arthrospores** and empty cells) in soil and **spherules** in tissue.
- Spherules are filled with endospores.
- Endemic in arid regions of Southern United States and Latin America.
- Bones and meninges commonly involved.
- Defect in cell-mediated immunity can result in disseminated diseases.
- Syndrome is called **'valley fever'** or **'desert rheumatism'**.
- May show **Erythema nodosum** (EN) **(desert bumps)**, which is delayed type hypersensitivity indicating good prognosis. There are no organisms in these lesions.
- Positive skin test with fungal extracts indicates good prognosis (good cell-mediated immunity). Negative skin test indicates risk or impending disseminated disease.
- Amphotericin B or itraconazole used for persisting lung lesions or disseminated disease.
- Fluconazole is drug of choice for meningitis.

### *Histoplasma*

- *Histoplasma capsulatum* causes histoplasmosis.

**in serum** and **chlamydospores** at ambient temperature on **Cornmeal** agar. It is a **polymorphic** fungus.

- Does not demonstrate thermal dimorphism.
- Germ tube formation, chlamydospore and pseudohyphae formation differentiate *C. albicans* from other *Candida* species.
- **Skin tests** with *Candida* antigens are used as an, **indicator of cellular immunity** and not for diagnosis. Negative *Candida* skin test means that the person is **anergic.**
- Drug of choice for oropharyngeal or esophageal thrush is fluconazole.
- Skin infections are treated with topical antifungals, e.g., clotrimazole or nystatin.
- Ketoconazole is used for mucocutaneous candidiasis.
- Disseminated candidiasis is treated with amphotericin B or fluconazole with or without flucytosine.
- Fluconazole is used for prevention of candidal infections in high-risk patients, like bone marrow transplantation.
- Nystatin "**swish and swallow**" or clotrimazole can be used to prevent oral thrush.

### *Cryptococcus*

- Belong to Phylum *Basidomycota.*
- *Cryptococcus neoformans* cause cryptococcosis, especially cryptococcal meningitis
- **Most common** life-threatening fungal disease in AIDS patients.
- Oval, budding **capsulated** yeast. Capsule is polysaccharide.
- **True yeast**, i.e. yeast at all temperatures/ conditions.
- **Narrow based bud** (unlike *Blastomyces*, which has broad based bud).
- Transmission of *Cryptococcus neoformans* var. *neoformans* occurs by **soil containing bird**

**(especially pigeon) droppings**. Birds do not suffer.

- *Cryptococcus neoformans* var. *gatti* is found in the **bark of eucalyptus trees**, commonly seen in North India.
- Human infection results from **inhalation**. No human to human transmission.
- Immunocompetent individuals can also be infected.
- Negative stain, **India ink,** on CSF shows capsulated yeasts. Meyer's **mucicarmine staining** shows pink capsule.
- Capsular antigen can be detected in CSF by **latex agglutination** test.
- Produces **urease** enzyme, can be grown on selective media like **niger seed agar** or **bird seed agar** where it forms black colonies.
- Amphotericin B and flucytosine used in meningitis. Fluconazole used for long-term suppression in AIDS patients.

## Aspergillus

- Belong to phylum ascomycota
- *Aspergillus fumigatus* causes infections of skin (wounds, burns), eyes (cornea), ears and other organs (paranasal sinuses); "**aspergilloma**" or "**fungus ball**" in the lungs (especially in lung cavities caused by tuberculosis) and allergic bronchopulmonary aspergillosis **(ABPA).** Most common cause of **fungal sinusitis**.
- Associated with immunocompromised, especially in neuropenia produces hemoptysis and granulomas
- Patients with ABPA show **asthmatic** symptoms, eosinophilia and high IgE titer against Aspergillus; expectorated bronchial plugs contain hyphae. Occupational asthma is associated with inhalation of conidia
- *Aspergillus flavus* grows on cereals or grains and forms **aflatoxin**, which is hepatotoxic and carcinogenic.

- Transmission by **airborne** conidia.
- **True molds** (exist only as hyphae); **septate** hyphae forming V-shaped **(dichotomous)** branches seen in tissue biopsy.
- Conidia present in **radiating chains** on a central stalk.
- High titers of **galactomannan** in invasive aspergillosis.
- Amphotericin B or caspofungin used against invasive aspergillosis.
- Fungal ball has to be surgical excision.
- ABPA treated with steroids and antifungals.

### Mucor and Rhizopus

- Belong to Phylum *Zygomycota.*
- Saprophytic molds that cause zygomycosis (or **mucormycosis**).
- Proliferate in the walls of **blood vessels** (predilection towards endothelial cells), result in thrombus formation that can lead to embolism and cause infarction of tissues distal to blocked vessel.
- **Diabetic ketoacidosis**, burns, leukemia are risk factors.
- Death due to disseminated intravascular coagulation **(DIC).**
- *Rhizopus oryzae* **commonest cause** of mucormycosis.
- **Coenocytic** (multinucleated, **nonseptate**) hyphae **branch at right angles.**
- *Rhizopus* forms **rhizoids**, mucor does not.
- Asexual spores are **sporangiospores** formed within sporangium.
- Treatment of underlying condition, amphotericin B and surgical excision of necrotic infected tissue.

### *Penicillium marneffii*

- **Dimorphic fungus** that causes tuberculosis-like disease in AIDS patients, especially **South East Asia**. India has both indigenous (northeast states like Manipur) and imported cases (across from Myanmar).

- *P. marneffii* is the only pathogenic and dimorphic member of genus *Penicillium.*
- Produces **rose colored pigment** at 25°C and not at 37°C.
- Demonstrates "**Corda's phenomenon**" (distal conidia are larger than those proximal to the vesicle, unlike other members of *Penicillium* or *Aspergillus*).
- Transmitted by **bamboo rats.**
- Culture and **Fluorescent antibody staining** of affected tissue done for diagnosis.
- Amphotericin B for 2 weeks followed by oral itraconazole for 10 weeks.

### *Pneumocystis carinii*

- Classified as a fungus (yeast related to *Saccharomyces cerevisiae*) on the **basis of molecular analysis** (rRNA sequences, mitochondrial DNA and enzymes), but medically many still consider as protozoan or unclassified.
- Does not grow on fungal media, antifungals not effective.
- Human species now called ***P. jiroveci*** (*P. carinii* is the rat species).
- Important cause of pneumonia in immunocompromised especially AIDS and premature infants.
- Transmission by **inhalation**, infection predominantly in lungs.
- Isolation of patients is not required.
- Sudden onset of fever, cough, dyspnoea and tachycardia is typical of pneumocystis; diffuse interstitial pneumonia.
- Cysts present in alveoli result in accumulation of plasma cells resulting in frothy exudate, known as **plasma cell pneumonia** (there is no invasion).
- Extrapulmonary infections in late stages of AIDS affect liver, spleen, lymph nodes and bone marrow.

- Mortality is 100% in untreated.
- Diagnosis by lung tissue from bronchoscopy, BAL or lung biopsy (sputum not suitable).
- Cysts can be seen with methenamine silver or Giemsa stain or Fluorescent-antibody staining (not Gram stain).
- **Non-cultivable organism** in culture.
- Trimethoprim-sulfamethoxazole (cotrimoxazole) drug of choice, pentamidine, atovaquone alternative drugs.

## PARAFUNGI

Organisms generically known as fungi, but not belonging to taxonomic Kingdom Fungi are known as parafungi. These are **hydrophilic** organisms unlike most fungi that are geophilic, anthropophilic or zoophilic.

### Important Parafungi

*Rhinosporidium seeberi*

- Causes **rhinosporidiosis** (benign, chronic inflammatory infection, manifests as **polyps** predominantly in **nasal** and upper respiratory sites.
- It is non-cultivable.
- Transmitted by water sources.
- Endospores and sporangia seen in the tissues.
- Splendore-Hoeppli phenomenon is not seen.

*Loboa loboi*

- Causes lobomycosis
- Transmission by dolphins.

*Pythium Insidiosum*

- Belongs to Kingdom *Chromista*, Phylum *Pseudo-fungi*.
- Organism of aquatic environment.
- Splendore-Hoeppli phenomenon is seen (eosinophilic infiltrates around lesions).

# CHAPTER FIVE

# Parasitology

- Parasites occur in two forms:
  - **protozoa** (single celled)
  - **helminthes** (multicellular).

| Important points to remember in parasites: |
|---|
| • infective form<br>• route of entry<br>• organ of localization<br>• invasive form<br>• portal of exit<br>• definitive host: host harboring sexual stage or adult forms intermediate host: host harboring asexual stage. |

## PROTOZOA

- Sarcodina (amoebae):
  - *Entamoeba histolytica*
  - *Naeglaria*
  - *Acantamoeba*
- Sporozoa
  - Coccidia:
    - *Cryptosporidium parvum*
    - *Isospora*
    - *Cyclospora*
  - Hematozoa:
    - *Plasmodium*
    - *Babesia*
    - *Toxoplasma*

- Mastigophora (flagellates):
  - *Giardia lamblia*
  - *Trichomonas*
  - Hemoflagellates
    - *Trypanosomes*
    - *Leishmania*
- Ciliophora (ciliates):
  - *Balantidium coli*
- Microspora (microsporidians):
  - *Enterocytozoon*
  - *Encepalitozoon*
  - *Nosema*
  - *Vittaforme cornea.*

## INTESTINAL AND UROGENITAL PROTOZOA

### *Entamoeba histolytica*

- Causes intestinal amoebiasis **(amoebic dysentery)** and extraintestinal amoebiasis **(liver abscess).**
- Two stages:
  - **cyst** (infective form): predominates in nondiarrhoeal stools, denotes chronicity/carrier, **killed by boiling but not by chlorination,** removed by filtration. Cyst has four nuclei (unlike eight in Entamoeba coli, nonpathogenic species).
  - **trophozoite** (invasive form): found in intestinal and extraintestinal lesions and in diarrhoeal stools, (only form found in tissues), **denotes acute** disease (presence of both trophozoites and cysts in the stool: acute on chronic), presence of RBCs inside is pathognomic.
- Transmitted by **feco-oral route** primarily (anal-oral in homosexuals), **no animal reservoir.**
- Typical **flask-shaped ulcer** in colon (unlike tubercular ulcers that are transverse leading to intestinal obstruction and typhoid ulcer that are longitudinal and lead to hemorrhage).

- May result in granulomatous lesion (**amoeboma**) in caecum or rectosigmoid colon that may look like adenocarcinoma.
- Aspiration of liver abscess yields brownish pus known as **anchovy sauce pus**, specimens taken from the edge of the abscess where trophozoites are found and not from necrotic center.
- Serologic testing is done for invasive amoebiasis: **IHA** (indirect haemagglutination).
- Culture can be done on Dobell's medium or Cleveland- Collier medium or NIH medium.
- Treatment of choice is metronidazole /tinidazole
- Asymptomatic cyst carriers treated with paromomycin or iodoquinol.

### *Giardia lamblia*

- Causes giardiasis.
- Infective form is **cyst**, invasive form is **trophozoite**
- Trophozoite is **pear-shaped**, with typical **tennis racket appearance, spoon like** concavity, **falling leaf motility.**
- Transmission by ingestion of cysts in fecally contaminated food and water.
- *Giardia* is the only common pathogenic protozoan found in duodenum and jejunum.
- Inflammation of duodenal mucosa and **malabsorption** of protein and fat.
- Cysts not killed by chlorination.
- Common in **homosexuals** due to oral-anal contact
- High incidence among children in **day care centers** and among patients in mental hospitals.
- **Non-bloody,** foul smelling diarrhea.
- Diagnose by finding trophozoites or cysts or both in stool.
- Only cysts seen in asymptomatic carriers.
- **String test** can be used if microscopy of stool in negative.
- Treatment by metronidazole.

### *Cryptosporidium parvum*

- Causes cryptosporidiosis, main symptom is diarrhea.
- Most severe in **immunocompromised,** e.g. AIDS.
- Acquired by feco-oral transmission of **oocysts.**
- **Jejunum** is most heavily infested.
- Invasion does not occur.
- Diagnosed by finding cysts in stool **by modified Kinyoun's acid-fast staining,** which is cold acid-fast staining.
- Oocysts are resistant to chlorination.

### *Trichomonas vaginalis*

- **Pear-shaped**, flagellated organism, which is a urogenital protozoa.
- Exists only as **trophozoite**, no cyst stage.
- Has an undulating membrane that extends for two-thirds of the length.
- Transmitted by **sexual contact.**
- Primary locations are **vagina** and prostate.
- Watery foul smelling **greenish vaginal discharge** with itching and burning.
- Usually asymptomatic in men, 10% may have urethritis.
- **Typical jerky motion** of trophozoites in vaginal or prostatic secretions.
- Metronidazole is drug of choice for both partners.

## BLOOD AND TISSUE PROTOZOA

### *Plasmodium*

- Causes malaria.
- Four important species:
  - *Plasmodium vivax* and *Plasmodium falciparum* are most important/common
  - *Plasmodium ovale* and *P. malariae* are uncommon.
- *P. malariae* causes quartan malaria (fever every fourth day) while others cause tertian malaria (fever every third day) if untreated.

- *P. malariae* infects only mature RBCs.
- People with sickle cell trait are protected from malaria.
- One of the most common infectious diseases and leading cause of death more than 200 million people worldwide have malaria and more than 1 million die each year.
- Transmitted by **female Anopheles** mosquito, which is the definite host and has sexual cycle; can also be transmitted across the placenta, in blood transfusion, and by intravenous drug abuse.
- Man is **intermediate host**, shows asexual cycle.
- Sexual cycle is called **sporogony**: sporozoites are produced in mosquito and transmitted to human by mosquito bite. Sporozoites are infective forms.
- Asexual cycle is called **schizogony**: schizonts are produced.
- Diagnosis is done by examination of peripheral blood smear; thick and thin film.
- **Thick film for diagnosing infection** and **thin film for differentiation of species.**
- If thick and thin film do not reveal parasites, ELISA for a specific protein of *P. falciparum* or PCR based test can be useful.

Life cycle

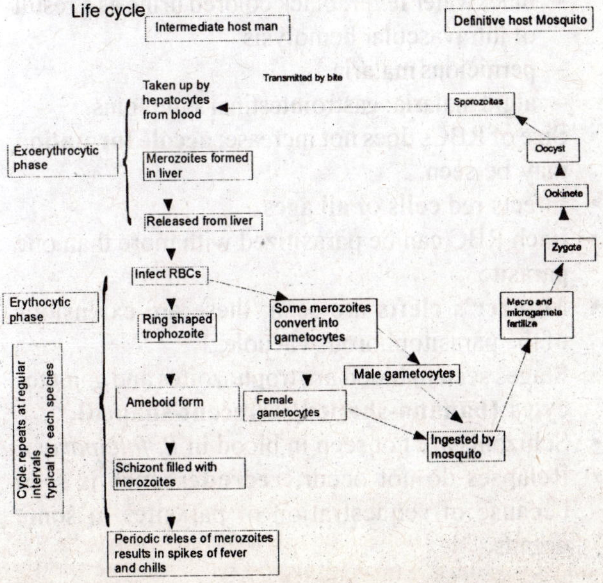

## Plasmodium vivax

- Causes benign tertian malaria, fever occurs every third day if untreated.
- Infects only reticulocytes (young RBCs).
- Size of RBCs is enlarged.
- **Schuffner's dots** are seen; these are indentations in the RBC membrane.
- Each RBC can have one parasite only.
- Stages seen in blood: Trophozoites (ring form, ameboid form), Gametocytes and Schizonts.
- Relapses are seen in *P. vivax*; as a result of fresh exoerythrocytic cycle in the liver caused by **hypnozoites**, latent form in the liver.
- People who are homozygous recessive for the genes that encode Duffy blood group are resistant to infection by *P. vivax*.

### *Plasmodium falciparum*

- Causes severe form of malaria.
- Causes malignant tertian malaria, fever occurs every fourth day if untreated.
- Causes complications like
  - cerebral malaria: also known as brain fever
  - blackwater fever: black colored urine as a result of intravascular hemolysis
  - pernicious malaria
  - algid malaria: gastrointestinal symptoms.
- Size of RBCs does not increase; **accolé formation** may be seen.
- Infects red cells of all ages.
- Each RBC can be parasitized with more than one parasite.
- **Maurer's clefts** are seen; these are extensions of the parasitophorous vacuole.
- Stages seen in blood are trophozoites and gametocytes **(banana-shaped/ crescent-shaped).**
- Schizonts are not seen in blood in *P. falciparum*.
- Relapses do not occur; **recrudescence** is seen because of sequestration of parasites in some organs.

- People with G6PD deficiency are also protected against severe effects of falciparum malaria.

**Treatment**

- **Chloroquine** is the drug of choice; chloroquine kills merozoites but not hypnozoites for which primaquine is effective, which must be used to prevent relapses.
- Most vivax are sensitive to chloroquine but many falciparum are found to be resistant to chloroquine. The percentage of resistant strains is increasing rapidly.
- For **chloroquine resistant strains** of *P. falciparum*, either mefloquine or a combination of quinine and doxycycline is used. Combination of atovaquone and proguanil is also available.

| Resistance to chloroquine is graded as: |
|---|
| **R1**: Low level resistance: Parasites disappear from blood after therapy but reappear usually within 7 days |
| **R2**: Intermediate level resistance: reduction of >75% followed by increase in number of parasites |
| **R3**: High-level resistance: Reduction of < 25% followed by increase in parasites |

**Chemoprophylaxis** for travelers to areas where malaria is endemic is chloroquine. Treatment should start 2 weeks before arrival and six weeks after departure followed by 2 weeks course of primaquine if the exposure was high.

Other preventive measures include use of mosquito nets, window screens, protective clothing and mosquito repellents.

***Toxoplasma gondii***

- Definitive host is domestic **cat,** humans are intermediate hosts.
- Ingestion of the cysts in undercooked meat or contact with cat feces.

- **Tachyzoites** (rapidly differentiated trophozoites) formed in the macrophages, kill cells and infect other cells, spread to brain, muscle and other tissues where they develop into slowly multiplying forms, **bradyzoites**. These are used for diagnosis in tissue specimen.
- In the cat, gametocytes are formed from bradyzoites in the gut and fuse to form oocysts that are excreted in cat feces.
- **Transplacental transmission** occurs by trachyzoites, other than this route human to human transmission does not occur.
- Cell-mediated immunity is important, but antibodies also play a role.
- **Congenital infection occurs only when mother is infected during pregnancy.**
- Congenital infection can result in abortion, stillbirth, encephalitis, chorioretinitis, hepatosplenomegaly, intracranial calcification.
- Congenital infection is an important cause of blindness in children.
- Life-threatening disseminated disease, mainly encephalitis occurs in immunocompromised (e.g. AIDS patients).
- Immunofluorescence for IgM antibody is used to diagnose acute and congenital infection (IgG can be maternal in origin).
- Significant rise of IgG titer in paired sera can also be used to diagnose acute infections.
- **Crescent-shaped trophozoites** in microscopic examination of Giemsa stained preparations.
- Cysts are seen in tissue.
- Can be grown in cell culture and confirmed in mice
- Congenital toxoplasmosis, disseminated disease in immunocompromised is treated with sulfadiazine and pyrimethamine.
- Prevention done by proper cooking of meat and avoidance of cats especially during pregnancy.

### Trypanosoma

Three major pathogens: ***T. cruzi, T. brucei gambiense, T. brucei rhodesiense.***

#### *Trypanosoma cruzi*

- Causes **Chaga's disease (American trypanosomiasis)**.
- Vector is **reduviid bug** (Triatoma, cone nose or kissing bug).
- Human and animals are reservoir hosts.
- Insects ingest **trypomastigotes** found in reservoir hosts, in insect gut, multiply, differentiate into epimastigotes and then into trypomastigote. These are deposited with feces on human skin when infected bug bites, then enters blood and converts into amastigote forms in host cells, which in turn convert into trypomastigote forms in blood.
- During acute phase, both trypomastigotes in blood and amastigote in tissue are seen. In chronic phase, only amastigote form is seen.
- Diagnosed by **demonstration of trypomastigotes in thick and thin films** (stained and wet preparations). Alternately, bone marrow aspirate or muscle biopsy (shows amastigotes); culture on special media; **xenodiagnosis**; serology: **indirect fluorescence antibody test** (earliest to become positive), indirect haemagglutination, complement fixation.
- **Myocardial** (most frequently and severely affected tissue), glial and reticuloendothelial cells are most frequent sites. Megacolon and megaesophagus are also seen.
- Death is due to cardiac arrhythmias and failure.
- Drug of choice is **nifurtimox** (more effective against trypomastigotes) for acute disease, alternative is benznidazole. No effective drug for chronic form. No vaccine.

- Chaga's disease occurs primarily in central and South America.
- Reduviid bug preferentially bites around the mouth or eyes (forms **chagoma**), hence called **kissing bug.**

*T. brucei (T. gambiense and T. rhodesiense)*

- Cause **sleeping sickness (African trypanosomiasis)**.
- Vector **is tsetse fly (** ***Glossina*****).**
- humans are reservoir for *T. gambiense*, whereas domestic animals and wild animals are reservoirs for *T. rhodesiense*.
- Infective form is **metacyclic trypomastigote** (transmitted by tsetse fly bite), which converts to blood form trypomastigotes, ingested by tsetse fly where they transform into epimastigotes and then into metacyclic trypomastigotes.
- Exhibit **antigenic variation** of surface glycoproteins, which is due to sequential movement of glycoprotein genes to a preferential location on the chromosome. These variations allow the organism to continually evade host immune response.
- Typical disease is **demyelinating encephalitis** presenting as somnolence (sleeping sickness).
- Endemic in sub-Saharan Africa.
- **Both sexes** of tsetse fly **can transmit** the disease.
- *T. gambiense* causes disease **along water courses** in west Africa, whereas *T. rhodesiense* is found **in arid regions** of east Africa.
- *T. gambiense* causes low grade chronic disease while *T. rhodesiense* causes acute, rapidly progressive disease fatal in months.
- Initial lesion is **"trypanosomal chancre"** at bite site; enlargement of cervical lymph nodes is common (**Winterbottom's sign**); encephalitis (progressing to somnolence and coma); death due to pneumonia in untreated cases.

- Microscopic examination of blood or aspirate from lymph node reveals **trypomastigotes;** presence in CSF indicates late encephalitic stage.
- Serology- ELISA for IgM.
- **Suramin,** drug of choice, must be initiated before encephalitis as it does not cross blood-brain barrier.
- Alternative is pentamidine. Suramin plus Melarsoprol is given for CNS symptoms.

### *Leishmania*

| | Old World Leishmaniasis | New World Leishmania |
|---|---|---|
| Agents: | *L. donovani, L. tropica, L. infantum* | *L. braziliensis, L. mexicana, L. panama* |
| Sandfly: | *Phlebotomus* | *Lutzomyia* |

### *Leishmania donovani*

- Cause of **kala azar** (Indian visceral leishmaniasis).
- **Sandfly**—Phlebotomus is the vector; only female flies are vectors.
- Sandfly transmits **promastigotes** (have flagellum with kinetoplast) which convert into **amastigote** {nonflagellated form—Leishman Donovan **(LD) bodies**} in the macrophages. Sandfly gets infected by eating macrophages containing amastigotes present in blood meal.
- **Reticuloendothelial** system (liver, spleen, and bone marrow) most severely affected.
- **Massive enlargement of the spleen** is seen; anemia, thrombocytopenia and leucopenia leading to secondary infections.
- **Hyperpigmentation** is characteristic (leading to term kala azar).
- **Bone marrow aspirate** is the specimen of choice; demonstration of LD bodies in bone marrow, spleen, lymph node or blood (**differential diagnosis**: *Histoplasma, P. marneffii*).
- Can be culture on **NNN** medium (Novy, Nicole, McNeal).

- Serology—**Indirect immunofluorescence** positive in most patients.
- **Leishmanin** skin test—negative during active disease but positive in recovered patients.
- Nonspecific tests for hypergammaglobulinemia-**antimony or aldehyde** test.
- **Sodium stibogluconate**, antimony compound is treatment of choice.
- Recovery results in immunity.

### *Leishmania tropica*

- Causes **Old World cutaneous leishmaniasis (Oriental sore, Delhi boil, Baghdad boil)**.
- Endemic in India, Middle East, Africa.
- Initial lesion is a papule at bite site, enlarges to form multiple nodules which coalesce and ulcerate. Heal in immunocompetent individuals but if cell-mediated immunity does not develop, spread to involve large areas of the skin with enormous numbers of organisms (analogous to tuberculosis and lepromatous leprosy).
- **Amastigotes** seen in smears taken from skin lesions.
- **Leishmanin** test positive when skin ulcer appears.
- Drug of choice is **sodium stibogluconate.**

### *Leishmania mexicana*

- Causes **New World cutaneous leishmaniasis (chicle ulcer, bay sore).**
- Found in Central and South America.

### *Leishmania braziliensis*

- Causes mucocutaneous leishmaniasis (**espundia**) and **American visceral leishmaniasis.**
- Occurs mostly in Brazil and Central America, mainly in **forestry and construction workers.**
- Lesions begin with papule at sandfly bite site, the metastatic lesions form usually at mucocutaneous junction of mouth and nose.

| *Organism* | *Vector stage* | *Infective stage* | *Invasive outside humans* | *Important stages* |
|---|---|---|---|---|
| *Plasmodium* | Female *Anopheles* mosquito | Sporozoite in mosquito saliva | Trophozoites and merozoites in RBCs | Mosquito ingests gametocytes- fuse to form zygote-ookinete-sporozoites |
| *Toxoplasma* | None | Tissue cyst (pseudocyst) in under-cooked meat or oocyst in cat feces | Tachyzoites (rapidly multiplying trophozoites, can pass placenta); bradyzoites are present in tissue cysts | Cat ingests tissue containing brady-zoites- gametes-ookinete- oocysts in feces |
| *Leishmania* | Sandfly (*Phlebo tomus* and *Lutzomyia*) | Promasti-gote in fly saliva | Amastigotes in macro-phages in liver spleen and bone marrow | Fly ingests macro-phages containing amastigotes-promastigotes |
| *Trypano-soma brucei* | Tsetse fly (*Glossina*) | Trypoma-stigote in fly saliva | Trypomas-tigotes in blood and brain | Fly ingests trypomastigote in human blood-epimastigote-trypomastigote |
| *Trypano-soma cruzi* | Reduviid bug (*Triatoma*) | Trypomas-tigote in bug feces | Amastigotes in cardiac muscle and neurons | Bug ingests trypomastigote in human blood-epimastigote-trypomastigote |

## MINOR PROTOZOAN PATHOGENS

### *Acanthamoeba* and *Naegleria*

- **Opportunistic amoebae or free living amoebae.**
- Cause meningoencephalitis, found in freshwater lakes or soil.
- Diagnosis made by amoebae in CSF.
- Prognosis is poor.
- Naegleria causes **primary amoebic meningo-encephalitis**, trophozoites enter while swimming; rapidly fatal, shows amoeboflagellate form.
- Acanthamoeba enters by trauma through skin or eyes, causes **granulomatous amoebic encephalitis**, primarily in immunocompromised.
- Acanthamoeba also causes **keratitis** associated with contact lens use.

- Another free living amoeba, ***Balamuthia,*** is rare and causes Acanthamoeba like meningoencephalitis.

### Babesia

- ***Babesia microti*** causes babesiosis, a zoonotic disease.
- Transmitted by bite of **tick, *Ixodes scapularis*** (same tick that transmits Lyme disease).
- **Sporozoite** in tick saliva is the infective form.
- *Babesia* **infects RBCs,** but unlike *Plasmodium* has no exoerythrocytic phase.
- Asplenic patients affected more severely.
- Diagnosed by microscopic examination of Giemsa stained blood smear.
- Typical "**Maltese Cross**" appearance in microscopy; no pigment in RBCs.
- Combined therapy with quinine and clindamycin.

### Balantidium

- ***B. coli*** is the **only ciliate to cause human disease.**
- Causes diarrhea.
- **Largest protozoan** to cause human disease.
- **Pigs** are main reservoirs.
- Human infected by **ingesting cysts.**
- **Trophozoites** are invasive form.
- No extraintestinal lesions are seen.
- Diagnosed by demonstrating large ciliated trophozoites or cysts with characteristic **V-shaped nucleus** in stool.

### Cyclospora

- ***Cyclospora cayetanensis*** is an intestinal protozoan.
- Causes watery diarrhea.
- Acquired by **feco-oral** transmission.
- No animal reservoir.
- **Prolonged and relapsing diarrhea** in immunocompromised.

- **Spherical oocysts** in modified acid-fast staining. of stool sample is diagnostic.
- Treatment of choice is **trimethoprim- sulfamethoxazole.**

## Isospora

- ***Isospora belli*** is an intestinal protozoan.
- Causes diarrhea especially in immunocompromised (**profuse watery diarrhea**) e.g. those with AIDS.
- **Oocyst** seen in stool.
- Treatment of choice is trimethoprim- sulfamethoxazole.

## HELMINTHS

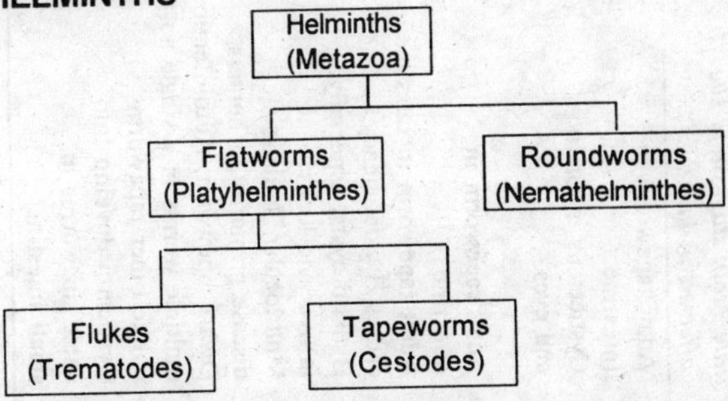


> Platyhelminthes are divided into two classes: Cestoda and Trematoda

### Cestodes (Tapeworms)

- Two main parts: scolex (head) and proglottids (segments)
- Scolex has suckers, hooks or sucking grooves
- Oldest proglottids are at the distal end and produce eggs that are excreted in the feces to be transmitted to intermediate hosts like cattle, pigs and fish
- Humans acquire infection when undercooked flesh containing larvae is ingested, however, in cysticercosis and hydatid disease, eggs are ingested and resulting larvae cause disease (Table 5.1).

### Trematodes

- Sexual cycle in humans and asexual reproduction in **freshwater snails (intermediate hosts)**.

**Table 5.1: Medically important cestodes**

| *Organism* | *Mode of transmission* | *Intermediate host(s)* | *Main stages and sites affected in humans* | *Diagnosis* | *Treatment* |
|---|---|---|---|---|---|
| *Taenia solium* | (A). ingest larvae in under-cooked pork | Pigs | Adult tapeworm in intestine | Proglottids in stool | Praziqantel |
| | (B). Ingest eggs in food or water contaminated with human feces | | Cysticercus in Brain and eyes | Biopsy, CT scan | Praziquantel or surgical removal of cysticerci |
| *Taenia saginata* | Ingest larvae in undercooked beef | Cattle | Adult tapeworm in intestine | Proglottids in stool | Praziquantel |
| *Diphyllobothrium latum* | Ingest larvae in undercooked fish | Copepods and Fish | Adult tapeworm in intestine; causes $B_{12}$ deficiency | Operculated eggs in stool | Praziquantel |
| *Echinococcus granulosus* | Ingest eggs in food contaminated with dog feces | Sheep, Human | Hydatid cysts, especially in liver and lungs | CT sacn, serology | Albendazole or surgical removal of cyst |
| *Echinococcus multilocularis* | Accidental ingestion of food contaminated with fox feces | Rodents | Multilocular hydatid disease primarily in hunters | CT scan | Albendazole or surgery |
| *Hymenolepis nana* | Ingested eggs are directly infectious | None | Dwarf tapeworm; Autoinfection; multiple worms in a single host unlike other tapeworms | Eggs in stool | Praziquantel |
| *Dipylidium caninum* | Occasionally infects humans when dog or cat fleas carrying cysticerci are ingested | | Cysticerci develop into adult tapeworms in small intestine | Typical barrel shaped proglottids in stool | Niclosamide |

- Transmission to humans takes place either by **penetration of skin** by free swimming cercaria of the schistosomes or **ingestion of cysts** in undercooked (raw) fish or crabs in *Clonorchis* and *Paragonimus* infection, respectively.
- Schistosomes (blood flukes) are **dieceous,** i.e. male and female are separate while other trematodes are hermaphrodite (**monoecious**).
- In most trematodes, Miracidium infect snails and cercaria infect humans.
- Treatment of choice is Praziquantel (Table 5.2).

### Nematodes (Roundworms)

- Cylindrical, asegmented body with complete digestive tract; rigid covering called cuticle.
- Nematodes have **separate sexes**; female is usually larger than the male.

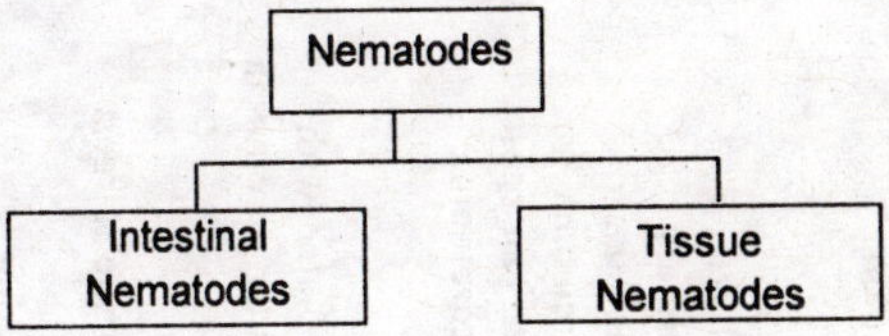


- Intestinal nematodes have two larval forms: first and second stage (**rhabditiform**) larvae are noninfectious, feeding forms; the third stage (**filariform**) larvae are the infectious, non-feeding forms.
- As adults, intestinal nematodes exist in the humans **except *Strongyloides***, which can also exist in the soil.
- *Ascaris, Trichuris, Taenia* have **bile stained eggs**, whereas *Enterobius*, hookworms and *H. nana* (cestode) have **non-bile stained eggs (Table 5.3).**
- Tissue nematodes are also known as **'filarial'** worms, because that produce motile embryos called microfilaria in blood or body fluids.

Table 5.2: Medically important trematodes

| *Organism* | *Transmission* | *Main Sites affected* | *Intermediate host* | *Diagnostic features of eggs* | *Endemic areas* |
|---|---|---|---|---|---|
| *Schistosoma mansoni* | Cercariae penetrate skin | Veins of colon | Snail | Large lateral spine | Africa, Latin America |
| *Schistosoma japonicum* | Cercariae penetrate skin | Veins of small intestine, liver | Snail | Small lateral spine | Asia |
| *Schistosoma haematobium* | Cercariae penetrate skin | Veins of urinary bladder; can lead to bladder carcinoma | Snail | Large terminal spine | Africa, Middle East |
| *Clonorchis sinensis* | Larvae in under-cooked fish | Biliary duct; can cause cholangiocarcinoma | Snail and fish | Operculated | Asia |
| *Paragonimus westermani* | Larvae in undercooked crab | Lung | Snail and crab | Operculated | Asia, India |
| *Fasciola hepatica* | Eating watercress (or other aquatic plants) contaminated with metacercaria (larvae) | Liver; associated with hepatocellular carcinoma | Snails | Eggs in stool | Latin America, Africa, Europe, China |
| *Fasciolopsis buski* | Eating aquatic vegetation contaminated with cysts | Small intestine (largest fluke) | Snails | Eggs in feces | Asia, India |
| *Heterophyes heterophyes* | Eating raw fish containing cysts | Small intestine | Snails | Eggs in feces | Africa, Middle East, Asia |

**Table 5.3:** Medically important intestinal nematodes

| *Organism* | *Common name or disease* | *Transmission* | *Diagnosis* | *Stage(s) in humans associated with disease* | *Important Stage(s) outside humans* | *Treatment* |
|---|---|---|---|---|---|---|
| *Enterobius vermicularis* | Pinworm, Seatworm | Ingestion of eggs | Eggs on perianal skin, no eggs in stool (NIH swab or Scotch tape used) | Female worm migrates out of anus and lays eggs on perianal skin, causing itching | None | Mebendazole or pyrantel pamoate |
| *Trichuris trichura* | Whipworm | Ingestion of eggs | Barrel-shaped (lemon-shaped) eggs in stool | Worms in colon may cause rectal prolapse | Eggs survive in environment | Mebendazole |
| *Ascaris lumbricoides* | Ascariasis (Roundworm) | Ingestion of eggs | Oval egg with irregular surface in stool | Largest intestinal nematodes; Larvae migrate to lung, causing Loeffler's pneumonia | Eggs survive in environment | Mebendazole or pyrantel pamoate |
| *Ancylostoma duodenale* (Old World hookworm) and *Necator americana* (New World hookworm) | Hookworm | Filariform larvae penetrate skin | Eggs in stool; eggs of *Ancylostoma* and *Necator* cannot be differentiated, adultworms needed for identification | Worms in colon cause blood loss (anemia) | Egg—rhabditiform larvae—filariform larvae | Mebendazole or pyrantel pamoate |

*Contd.*

*Contd.*

| | | | | | | |
|---|---|---|---|---|---|---|
| *Strongyloides stercoralis* | Strongyloidiasis | Filariform larvae penetrate skin; also autoinfection | Larvae in stool | Worms disseminate in various tissues in immunocompromised (autoinfection); Eosinophilia | Egg→ rhabditiform larvae→ filariform larvae; also free living cycle in soil | Ivermectin |
| *Trichinella spiralis* | Trichinosis | Larvae in undercooked meat (especially pigs) | Larvae encysted in muscle, serology | Larvae encyst in (striated) muscle causing myalgia; humans are 'end stage' hosts; subconjunctival hemorrhage, periorbital edema | Larvae in muscle of pig, other animals | Thiabendazole for adultworms |
| *Anisakis simplex* | Anisakiasis | Larvae in undercooked seafood (fish) | Clinical | Larvae in submucosa of GI tract | Adultworm in whales, dolphins; adults produce eggs that are eaten by crustaceans which are eaten by marine fish; Larvae in fish muscle | No drug available |
| *Gnathostoma spinigerum* | Meningitis | Eating undercooked fish | Clinical; demonstration of larvae in CSF | Larvae in CSF | Intestine of cats and dogs | Albendazole |

**Table 5.4:** Medically important trematodes

| *Organism* | *Common name or Disease* | *Transmission* | *Diagnosis* | *Stage(s) in human associated with* | *Treatment* |
|---|---|---|---|---|---|
| *Wuchereria bancrofti* | Bancroftian filariasis (elephantiasis) | Larvae transmitted by Mosquito bite (female Anopheles or Culex) | Microfilaria (tail tip free of nuclei, sheathed) in blood smear | Adult worms in lymphatics cause blockage | Diethyl carbamazine |
| *Brugia malayi* | Brugian filariasis | Larvae transmitted by Mosquito bite (female Culex) | Microfilaria (two nuclei in tail tip; sheathed) in blood smear | Adult worms in lymphatics | Diethyl carbamazine |
| *Loa loa* | Loiasis | Larvae transmitted by Deerfly (mangofly), *Chrysops*, bite | Microfilaria (nuclei fill tail tip; sheathed) in blood smear | Adult worm in tissue (skin, conjunctivae); adult worm crawling across conjunctiva) | Diethyl carbamazine |
| *Onchocerca volvulus* | Onchocerciasis (river blindness) | Larvae transmitted by female Blackfly (*Simulium*) bite | Skin biopsy | Adult worm in skin; microfilaria (unsheathed) in eye (blindness); hanging groin; lizard skin | Ivermectin |

*Contd.*

*Contd.*

| | | | | | |
|---|---|---|---|---|---|
| *Dracunculus medinensis* | Guinea worm | Ingestion of larvae in crustaceans (copepods) in contaminated drinking water | Clinical; head of female worm appears from a skin ulcer to lay down eggs | Female worms cause skin blister | Thiabendazole prior to extracting worm by winding it up on a stick over days |
| *Toxocara* (*T. canis* or *T. cati*) larvae | Visceral larva migrans | Ingestion of eggs in dog or cat feces | Clinical and serologic; larvae in tissue | Larvae in internal organs liver, brain; or eyes; blindness most serious finding | Albendazole or mebendazole |
| *Ancylostoma* (*A. caninum* or *A. braziliense*) larvae | Cutaneous larva migrans | Filariform larvae penetrate skin; life cycle cannot be completed in humans | Clinical | Larvae in subcutaneous tissue; creeping eruption | Thiabendazole |
| *Angio-strongylus cantonensis* | Eosinophilic meningitis | Eating undercooked seafood | Clinical; occasionally demonstration of larvae in CSF | Larvae in spinal fluid; Rat lung nematode | None |

- Tissue nematodes are transmitted from person to person by **insect bite** (mosquito or flies) except guinea worm (*Dracunculus*), whose larvae inhabit crustaceans and are **ingested** in drinking water.
- Most nematodes cause disease due to presence of adultworms in human body; in some, larvae can cause disease like **visceral larva migrans** caused by larvae of *Toxocara canis*, **cutaneous larva migrans** caused by *Ancylostoma caninum* larvae.

## CHAPTER SIX

# Virology

### Viruses

- Are composed of **either DNA or RNA (not both)** covered by a protective protein coat (capsid), together called nucleocapsid.
- Nucleocapsid may have helical or icosahedral symmetry.
- **Do not have a nucleus, cytoplasm, mitochondria, or ribosomes.**
- May be enveloped (lipoprotein—lipid derived from host and protein is virus specific) or non-enveloped.
- **Are obligate intracellular pathogens.**

| All helical human viruses are enveloped, i.e. there are no naked helical viruses. |
|---|

Viruses show host and organ specificity and they are highly antigenic. Some viruses produce superantigens, **Herpesviruses**—Epstien Barr and CMV, and **Retrovirus**—mouse mammary tumor virus.

> Complete viral particle is known as virion
>
> Atypical virus like agents:
>
> - Defective viruses : cannot replicate without helper virus
> - Pseudovirus: contains host DNA instead of viral DNA in the capsid
> - Viroids: single molecule of circular RNA without protein coat or envelope
> - Prions: composed solely of protein, no detectable nucleic acid, cause transmissible. Spongiform encephalopathy.

## Viral Growth Cycle

Attachment (specificity of attachment determines host range of virus)→Penetration→Uncoating→Gene expression→ Genome Replication→ Assembly→ Release.

**Classification** of viruses is based on chemical and morphologic criteria:

- Nucleic acid: size and structure.
- Capsid: size, symmetry, and whether it is enveloped.

> All DNA viruses, except poxviruses, replicate in the nucleus.
> All RNA viruses, except retroviruses and influenza, replicate in the cytoplasm.
> All DNA viruses have double-stranded genome except parvoviruses, which have single-stranded DNA.
> All RNA viruses have single-stranded genome except reoviruses, which have double-stranded RNA.
> Enveloped viruses can infect by parenteral route only.

Classification of virus families causing human infections

| *Nucleic acid* | *Capsid symmetry* | *Enveloped or naked* | *Ether sensitivity* | *Strands* | *Virus family* |
|---|---|---|---|---|---|
| **DNA** | Icosahedral | Naked | Resistant | ss | Parvoviridae |
| | | | | ds circular | Polyomaviridae |
| | | | | ds circular | Papillomaviridae |
| | | | | ds | Adenoviridae |
| | | Enveloped | Sensitive | ds partial, circular | Hepadnaviridae |
| | | | | ds | Herpesviridae |
| | Complex | Complex coats | Resistant | ds | Poxviridae |
| **RNA** | Icosahedral | Naked | Resistant | ss | Picornaviridae |
| | | | | ss | Astroviridae |
| | | | | ss | Caliciviridae |
| | | | | ds segmented | Reoviridae |
| | | Enveloped | Sensitive | ss | Togaviridae |
| | | | | ss | Flaviviridae |
| | Unknown or complex | Enveloped | Sensitive | ss segmented | Arenaviridae |
| | | | | ss | Coronaviridae |
| | | | | ss diploid | Retroviridae |
| | | | | ss segmented | Orthomyxoviridae |
| | Helical | Enveloped | Sensitive | ss segmented | Bunyaviridae |
| | | | | ss | Bornaviridae |
| | | | | ss | Rhabdoviridae |
| | | | | ss | Paramyxoviridae |
| | | | | ss | Filoviridae |

## Diagnosis of Viral Diseases

1. **Identification of the virus in cell culture**:
   - Growth of virus in cell culture may produce a characteristic **cytopathic effect** (CPE) that can provide a presumptive identification.
   - CPE can be in the form of changes in the shape, size, and fusion of cells to form multinucleate giant cell.
   - Time taken to produce CPE and type of cells involved are also important for diagnosis.
   - If a virus does not produce CPE, it may be detected in cell culture by **haemadsorption** (e.g. for mumps, influenza virus), **interference** with formation of CPE by a second virus (e.g. rubella virus, which is detected by interference with the formation of CPE by echovirus or coxsackie virus).
   - **Definitive identification** of virus grown in cell culture is made by using known antibody in tests like
     - Complement fixation,
     - Hemagglutination inhibition,
     - Neutralization of CPE
     - Fluorescent antibody
     - Radioimmunoassay
     - ELISA
     - Immunoelectron microscopy.

> Viruses can be **grown by**:
> - **Inoculation in animals**: Susceptible animal has to be chosen. This may not always be possible. Not a method for routine diagnosis.
> - **Embryonated eggs:** Common method used prior to discovery of cell cultures. Hen's embryonated eggs most commonly used. Parts of egg used for viral growth:
>   - Amniotic cavity: for primary isolation of viruses from specimen
>   - Yolk sac: for vaccine production

- Allantoic cavity: for raising antigens for diagnostic kits or research purposes
- Chorioallantoic membrane: differentiate viruses on the basis of type of pocks produced; differentiation of variola and vaccinia (poxviruses); HSV1 and HSV2 (herpesviruses)

- **Cell cultures**: could be in the form of:
  - Monolayers: single layer of one type of cells grown *in vitro*:
    - **Primary cell culture:** for primary isolation from specimen
    - **Diploid or semicontinuous cell culture:** for vaccine production; can be subcultured for not more than 20-50 times
    - **Continuous cell lines:** for antigen production for diagnostic kits or research purposes; derived from malignant cells, therefore can be subcultured indefinitely, e.g. HeLa cell line derived from carcinoma cervix cells is still used after 60 years of origin.
  - **Organ/Tissue/Explant culture:** a tissue or a part of an organ with multiple cell types and architecture maintained, e.g. tracheal ring culture done for coronaviruses.

2. **Microscopic identification** directly in the specimen:
   - *Light microscopy:* can show inclusion bodies (viral replication sites) or multinucleate giant cells, e.g. Tzank smear for Herpes virus.
   - *UV microscopy:* used for fluorescent antibody staining of virus in infected cells.
   - *Electron microscopy:* detects virus particles, which can be differentiated by size and morphology.

2. **Serologic procedures** to detect a four-fold rise in antibody titer between acute phase and convalescent phase samples (taken 10-14 days apart) or the presence of IgM antibody. In some cases like infectious mononucleosis, heterophile antibody tests are also used.

3. **Detection of viral antigens** in blood or body fluids mostly done by ELISA; e.g. p24 antigen of HIV; HBsAg of Hepatitis B.
4. **Detection of viral nucleic acids** in blood or patient's cells either by using complementary DNA or RNA as a probe; or by amplification using PCR.

# DNA VIRUSES

## DNA NONENVELOPED VIRUSES

### Parvoviruses

- Parvovirus B19 causes erythema infectiosum (slapped cheek syndrome, **fifth disease**), **aplastic anemia** (especially in patients with **sickle cell anemia**) and fetal infections **(hydrops fetalis).**
- Has a single stranded DNA genome, icosahedral symmetry .
- Has only one serotype.
- Replication occurs in the nucleus; single-stranded DNA has **'hairpin' loops** at both ends which allow cellular DNA polymerase to initiate replication.
- B19 virus replicates only when a cell is in S phase, therefore it replicates in red cell precursors but not mature red cells; also infects endothelial cells.
- Transmitted by respiratory route; also trans-placentally or by blood transfusions.
- Diagnosed by detecting IgM antibodies or by PCR analysis.

### Papillomaviruses

- Cause papillomas, which are benign tumors of skin (e.g. warts or **condylomata acuminata**) or carcinomas, especially carcinoma of cervix and penis.
- Nonenveloped viruses with double-stranded circular DNA and icosahedral symmetry.
- Two genes E6 and E7 are implicated in carcinogenesis.
- More than 100 types of papillomaviruses classified on the basis of DNA restriction fragment analysis.

- Skin warts caused mainly by HPV 1-4, genital warts usually caused by HPV 6 and 11.
- Carcinomas and premalignant condition intraepithelial neoplasia associated with HPV 16 and 18.
- Transmitted by skin-to-skin contact and genital contact.
- **Koilocytes** (vacuolated cells) are characteristic of infection.
- Usually diagnosed clinically; presence of koilocytes indicates HPV infection; DNA hybridization tests also available.
- Treatment of genital warts is podophyllin; liquid nitrogen for skin warts; cidofovir is severe HPV infections.

## POLYOMAVIRUSES

### JC virus

- Causes **Progressive Multifocal Leucoencephalopathy.**
- **BK virus:** Causes renal infection and transplant rejection.

### Adenoviruses

- Cause upper and lower respiratory tract infections like pharyngitis, conjunctivitis, common cold, pneumonia.
- Also cause **keratoconjunctivitis, hemorrhagic cystitis and gastroenteritis;** cause sarcomas in rodents.
- Nonenveloped, isosahedral symmetry.
- These are the only viruses with a fiber protruding from each of the vertices of the capsid; this is the organ of attachment and is a haemagglutinin and toxic to humans.
- Adenoviruses have 41 serotypes; e.g. type 3, 4, 7, 21 cause respiratory disease; **type 8 and 19** cause epidemic keratoconjunctivitis; **type 11 and 21** cause hemorrhagic cystitis; and **type 40, 41** cause infantile gastroenteritis.

- After replication, viruses are released by lysis of the cell, not budding.
- Transmitted by aerosol droplet, feco-oral route an direct inoculation of conjunctivas.
- Diagnosis by isolation in cell culture and serology (CFT, haemagglutination inhibition).

## DNA ENVELOPED VIRUSES

### Herpesviruses

Common human herpes viruses (HHV)

HHV 1: Herpes simplex virus (HSV) 1
HHV 2: HSV 2
HHV 3: Varicella zoster virus (VZV)
HHV 4: Ebstein-Barr virus (EBV)
HHV 5: Cytomegalovirus (CMV)
HHV 6: Roseola infantum virus (sixth disease, exanthema septicum)
HHV 7: Human herpes virus 7
HHV 8: Kaposi sarcoma associated virus (KSAV).

- Herpesviruses show icosahedral symmetry.
- Second largest viruses (after Poxviruses).
- Replicate in the nucleus forming intranuclear inclusion bodies.
- Only viruses that obtain their envelopes by **budding from the nuclear membrane.**
- Ability to cause latent infections.
- Three subdivisions:
  - Alpha herpesviruses: HSV1, HSV 2, VZV infect epithelial cells primarily and cause latent infection in neurons
  - Beta herpesviruses: CMV, HHV 6, infect an become latent in a variety of tissues
  - Gamma herpes viruses: EBV, HHV 8, infect and become latent primarily in lymphoid cells.

### Herpes Simplex Viruses

- HSV-1 causes lesions **'above the waist' (acute gingivostomatitis, recurrent herpes labialis** (cold sores), **keratitis**, and **encephalitis**; **Herpetic whitlow** in medical personnel as a result of contact).

- HSV-2 causes lesions '**below the waist**' (genital herpes), also neonatal herpes (ranging from severe disease like encephalitis to mild local lesions) and aseptic meningitis when acquired at the time of birth during passage through infected mother's birth canal.
- HSV-1 is transmitted mainly in saliva, whereas HSV-2 is transmitted by sexual contact.
- Virus replicates in the skin or mucous membrane, then migrates up the neuron and becomes latent in the sensory ganglion cells; **HSV-1 in trigeminal ganglia, HSV-2 in sacral ganglia.** Virus can be reactivated by various inducers, e.g. sunlight, hormonal changes, stress, fever, at which time the virus migrates down the neuron and replicates in the skin, causing lesions.
- Typical skin lesion is a vesicle that has serous fluid full of virus particles. The vesicles may rupture and virus gets transmitted to others.
- Multinucleate giant cells are typically found at the base of lesions.
- Reactivation and reinfection are seen.
- Laboratory diagnosis.
  - Isolation in cell culture: typical cytopathic effects in 1-3 days.
  - Rapid diagnosis by **Tzanck smear** from skin lesions (stained by Giemsa stain).
  - Rapid diagnosis of encephalitis by detecting HSV-1 DNA in spinal fluid by PCR.
  - Neonatal herpes diagnosed by use of viral cultures or PCR assay.
  - Serologic test such as neutralization test for primary infections.
- Treatment
  - Acyclovir is the treatment of choice for encephalitis and systemic disease by HSV-1.

  - Also used for primary and recurrent genital herpes; shortens the durations and reduces the extent of shedding.
- No effect on the latent stage but prophylaxis can prevent recurrences.
- Prevention
  Cesarean section is recommended for infected expectant mothers at term.

### Varicella Zoster Virus (VZV)

- Varicella **(chickenpox)** is the primary disease; herpes zoster **(shingles)** is the recurrent form.
- Has a single serotype.
- Transmitted by respiratory droplets and direct contact.
- There is infectious VZV in zoster vesicles; can be transmitted by direct contact to children and cause chickenpox.
- Typical lesion is vesicular rash (in chickenpox, rash appears on trunks first. Zoster appears along the path of a sensory nerve of head or trunk) .
- **Multinucleate giant cells** with intranuclear inclusions seen in the base of the lesions.
- After recovery, virus becomes latent in dorsal root ganglia.
- Later in life, reactivation can lead to vesicular lesions and nerve pain of zoster.
- **Immunity after varicella is lifelong** but zoster can occur despite immunity to varicella. Zoster usually occurs only once.
- Diagnosis is almost always made clinically, although virus can be demonstrated from the lesions.
- Acyclovir, Famciclovir, Valacyclovir can reduce the severity and duration, although they cannot cure the latent stage and do not have any effect on post-herpetic neuralgia.
- Vaccine is a live, attenuated VZV **(Oka strain)**. Prevents chickenpox but not zoster in people who have already suffered from chickenpox.

- Should not be given to immunocompromised people or pregnant women.

**Cytomegalovirus (CMV)**

- Causes **cytomegalic inclusion disease** (especially congenital abnormalities) in neonates.
- Also causes **pneumonia** and **retinitis** in immunocompromised; **infectious mononucleosis like disease** in immunocompetent.
- Has a single serotype.
- Transmission:
  - Early in life
    - Transplacental
    - Within the birth canal
    - Breast milk.
  - In young children via saliva.
  - Later in life transmitted sexually (semen, cervical secretions).
  - Can also be transmitted during blood transfusions and organ transplants.
  - Congenital infections are more common if fetus is infected during the first trimester; may present as **microcephaly**, seizures, deafness, mental retardation, hepatosplenomegaly.
  - Infections in children and adults are generally asymptomatic, except in immunocompromised
  - CMV retinitis may be the first sign of AIDS related illnesses.
  - Can be cultured in 'shell vial' culture.
  - Intranuclear inclusion bodies have an oval **owl's eye shape** and can be seen with histologic staining in giant cells in urine and in tissue.
  - PCR based assays in tissue or body fluids like spinal fluid or amniotic fluid.
  - Gancyclovir is effective in treatment of CMV retinitis and pneumonia in AIDS patients.
  - Fomivirsen for intraocular treatment of CMV retinitis.
  - Blood for transfusion to newborns and organs from donors for transplantation should be CMV negative.

### Epstein Barr Virus (EBV)

- Causes **infectious mononucleosis.**
- Associated with **Burkitt's lymphoma,** other **B cell lymphomas**, and **nasopharyngeal carcinoma.**
- Also associated with hairy leukoplakia, a non-malignant lesion on tongue especially in AIDS.
- Most important antigen is viral capsid antigen (VCA), used in diagnosis; other antigens are early antigen (EA) and EBNA (nuclear antigen).
- Mainly infects B lymphocytes.
- Transmitted by exchange of saliva; known as **kissing disease.**
- IgM antibodies to VCA is used to diagnose acute infection.
- Non-specific heterophile antibodies (Monospot test) are also used for diagnosis.

### Human Herpes Virus 8 (Kaposi Sarcoma Associated Herpes Virus)

- Associated with Kaposi Sarcoma, **the most common cancer in AIDS.**
- Transmission of HHV-8 is primarily sexual, but is also transmitted in transplanted organs like kidneys and results in transplantation associated Kaposi sarcoma.
- Malignancy of vascular endothelial cells that contain many spindle-shaped cells and erythrocytes.
- Dark purple, flat to nodular lesions on skin, oral cavity and soles (but not palms)
- Also infect B cells to produce primary effusion lymphoma
- Laboratory diagnosis is made by biopsy of skin lesions. Important differential diagnosis is bacillary angiomatosis caused by *Bartonella bacilliformis*.

## POXVIRUSES

Largest and most complex viruses:

Different members have specificity for different types of hosts, e.g. orthopox, parapox, avipox, molluscipox.

### Smallpox Virus

- Known as **Variola virus.**
- Only disease that has been eradicated from Earth.
- **Brick-shaped** with double-stranded DNA.
- Virus contains a DNA-dependent RNA polymerase as it belongs to the only DNA virus group that **replicates in the cytoplasm.**
- Single stable serotype that is the key to the success of vaccine.
- Infects only humans, there is no animal reservoir.
- Transmitted via aerosol or direct contact.
- Last naturally occurring case was in Somalia in 1977.
- Incubation period in 7-14 days; rash is worse on face and extremities (centrifugal distribution).
- Diagnosis used to be made by growing virus in cell culture or chick embryos or by detecting viral antigens in vesicular fluid by immunofluorescence.
- Disease was eradicated by use of live attenuated vaccinia virus vaccine.
- Vaccine inoculated intradermally.
- Immunization now done in military personnel due to possibility of use of smallpox virus in biological warfare.
- In a bioterrorism event with smallpox virus, 'ring immunization' of general public could be undertaken as an exposed individual can be immunized as long as 4 days after exposure and be protected.

### Molluscum Contagiosum Virus

- Member of poxvirus family, causes small, pink, wart-like benign tumors of the skin or mucous membranes.
- Lesions have a characteristic cup-shaped crater with a white core.

- Transmitted by close personal contact, including sexually.
- Diagnosis is made clinically; virus cannot be grown in cell culture **(non-cultivable virus).**
- Removal of lesion by curettage or with liquid nitrogen may be effective.

### Hepatitis B virus

- Hepatitis B, an enveloped DNA virus, is described with other Hepatitis viruses.

## RNA ENVELOPED VIRUSES

### ORTHOMYXOVIRUSES

#### Influenza viruses

- These are the only members of orthomyxoviridae
- Negative sense viruses; contain RNA-dependent RNA polymerase
- Segmented single-stranded enveloped RNA viruses, helical symmetry
- Two types of spikes: **haemagglutination and neuraminidase.**
- Influenza A causes pandemics of influenza; Influenza B causes outbreaks; Influenza C causes mild respiratory infections but no outbreaks
- Show changes in antigenicity which can be:
  - **antigenic shift:** major changes based on reassortment of segments
  - **antigenic drift:** minor changes based on mutations in RNA genome
- Antibody against hemagglutinin neutralizes the infectivity of the virus and prevents disease
- Many species of animals have their own influenza A viruses. These animal viruses are the source of the segments that result in antigenic shift, e.g. if avian and human influenza A virus in the same cell, reassortment could occur and a new variant of human A virus may appear.

- H1N1 and H3N2 are most common; H2N2 caused a pandemic in 1968.
- In 1997, a new strain, **H5N1**, previously limited to chickens, resulted in human disease in Hong Kong.
- In 2003-2004, human deaths were reported; human to human transmission is poor but reassortment could change this leading to catastrophic results.
- Influenza viruses have an important stage of their replication take place in the nucleus.
- Transmitted by airborne respiratory droplets; occurs primarily in winter months.
- Virus can be detected in nasal or throat washings, nasal or throat swabs, and sputum by various techniques like direct fluorescent antibody, PCR, or cell culture-based tests.
- Can also be diagnosed by detection of antibodies in serum by hemagglutination inhibition or complement fixation test.
- **Amantadine** is used for treatment and prevention of influenza A; Zanamivir and oseltamivir are also used (neuraminidase inhibitors).
- **Vaccine is reformulated each year** to contain current antigenic strains.
- Two types of vaccines: killed and live attenuated are available. Killed provides immunity for 6 months and low mucosal immunity.
- Live attenuated provides mucosal immunity also and is administered by intranasal route.

## PARAMYXOVIRUSES

- Contains four important human pathogens:
  - **Measles virus, mumps virus, respiratory syncytial virus, parainfluenza viruses.**
- Not segmented, i.e. composed of one piece of single-stranded RNA (unlike orthomyxoviruses), enveloped and show helical symmetry.
- Contain RNA dependent RNA polymerase; as they have negative polarity.

### Measles Virus

- Causes measles.
- Single serotype; humans are natural hosts.
- Transmitted via respiratory droplets during prodromal period and few days after rash appears.
- Rash is caused by cytotoxic T cells attaching measles virus infected vascular endothelial cells in the skin. Shortly after the rash appears, virus can no longer spread to others.
- **Multinucleated giant cells** are characteristic of the lesions. Inclusion bodies seen both intranuclear and intracytoplasmic.
- Lifelong immunity following the disease.
- Infants are protected during first 6 months of life as a result of maternal antibody passing through the placenta.
- **Koplik's spots** are diagnostic; these are bright red lesions with white central dot on the buccal mucosa.
- Maculopapular rash appears on the face and proceeds down the body to lower extremities, including palms and soles.
- Complications include encephalitis, deafness, mental retardation, pneumonia, bacterial otitis media and **subacute sclerosing panencephalitis (SSPE).**
- Increased risk of stillbirth in pregnant women.
- Most diagnoses are made on clinical features, but virus can be isolated in cell culture; rise in antibody titer can also be used for diagnosis.
- **Live, attenuated vaccine** is effective; given subcutaneously (at 9 months in India followed by a combination vaccine with rubella and mumps at 15 months of age).
- Should not be given to immunocompromised individuals and pregnant women.

### Mumps Virus

- Causes mumps.

- Single serotype.
- Humans are natural hosts.
- Transmitted via respiratory droplets.
- Occurs more in winters.
- About 30% children have subclinical infection, which provides immunity.
- Infects the parotid gland, testes, ovaries, pancreas and rarely meninges.
- **Lifelong immunity after disease.**
- Protection in first 6 months by maternal antibodies.
- Complications include **orchitis** in postpubertal males, which can lead to sterility, and meningitis, which is usually self-limiting.
- Diagnosis is usually made clinically; virus can be isolated in cell culture from saliva, spinal fluid, or urine.
- Serology by haemagglutination inhibition or CFT is diagnostic.
- Mumps skin test is used to determine whether a patient's cell-mediated immunity is competent.
- **Live attenuated vaccine** is effective; given subcutaneously at 15 months of age in combination with measles and rubella.
- Should not be given to immunocompromised individuals or pregnant women.

### Respiratory Syncytial Virus

- Most important cause of **bronchiolitis in infants;** also important in pneumonia; in older children causes otitis media; in adults resembles common cold.
- Its surface spikes are **fusion proteins,** which cause cells to fuse forming multinucleate giant cells **(syncytia),** which gives rise to the name of this virus.
- Humans and chimpanzees are natural hosts.
- Transmission occurs via **respiratory droplets** and by direct contact of contaminated hands with nose or mouth.

- Causes outbreaks every winter; also outbreaks in hospitalized infants.
- Outbreaks can be controlled by hand washing and use of gloves.
- Infection in infants is more severe; infection does not provide immunity.
- Virus can be detected rapidly by **immunofluorescence** on smears of respiratory epithelium or by isolation in cell culture.
- Cytopathic effect is formation of **multinucleate giant cells**; serology is also diagnostic.
- **Aerosolized ribavirin** is recommended for severely ill hospitalized infants; combination of ribavirin and hyperimmune globulins may be more effective.

### Parainfluenza Viruses

- Cause **croup** (acute laryngotracheobronchitis), laryngitis, bronchitis, and pneumonia in children and common cold like symptoms in adults.
- Transmitted via respiratory droplets.
- Disease occurs mainly in winters.
- Parainfluenza 1 and 2 major causes of croup.
- Croup is characterized by a harsh cough and hoarseness.
- Mostly diagnosed clinically; virus can be isolated in cell culture or serology can be done for 4-fold rise in antibody titer.

### Hendra Virus

- First identified as human pathogen in 1994, caused severe respiratory disease in Hendra, Australia.
- Acquired by contact with horses.

### Nipah Virus

- Paramyxovirus caused encephalitis in Malaysia and Singapore in 1998 and 1999.
- A major outbreak of encephalitis in Siliguri in West Bengal in 2001 has now been proven to be caused by Nipah virus.

## CORONAVIRUSES

- Important cause of common cold, second to rhinoviruses.
- In 2002, a new disease, an atypical pneumonia called **SARS** (Severe acute respiratory syndrome) emerged.
- Nonsegmented, single-stranded, positive sense, enveloped viruses with helical symmetry.
- In electron microscopy, prominent club-shaped spikes in the form of **'corona; (halo)** can be seen.
- Two serotypes 229E and OC43.
- Common cold caused by coronaviruses has no long-term sequelae.
- SARS virus (CoV-SARS) is different from existing human coronaviruses.
- Virus obtains its envelop from the endoplasmic reticulum, not from plasma membrane.
- Transmitted by respiratory aerosol. SARS originated in China in November 2002 and spread to other countries. Fatality rate has been 9%. Human to human transmission occurs and some patients are thought to be 'super-spreaders'. Early in the outbreak hospital personnel were affected, but respiratory infection control procedures have reduced spread within hospitals.
- **Civet cat** appears to be the likely reservoir of CoV-SARS.
- SARS is a severe atypical pneumonia characterized by high-grade fever, nonproductive cough, dyspnea and hypoxia. Chest X-ray reveals interstitial 'ground glass' infiltrates that do not cavitate. Incubation ranges from 2 to 10 days.
- If SARS is suspected, antibody based and PCR based tests can be used.

## TOGAVIRUSES

### Rubella virus

- Causes rubella **(German measles)** and congenital rubella syndrome.

- Icosahedral symmetry, enveloped, positive strand RNA.
- **Single antigenic type.**
- Transmitted via respiratory droplets and from mother to fetus transplacentally.
- Natural infection leads to lifelong immunity.
- Antibody crosses the placenta and protects the newborn.
- Rubella is milder, shorter disease than measles. Incubation of 14-21 days is followed by a maculopapular rash, which starts on the face and progresses downward to involve extremities. Post-auricular lymphadenopathy is common. Rash typically lasts 3 days. Could be accompanied by polyarthritis in adults.
- When a nonimmune pregnant woman is infected during the **first trimester, especially first month,** significant congenital malformations can occur, e.g. patent ductus arteriosus, cataracts, deafness and mental retardation.
- Some children infected *in utero* can continue to excrete rubella virus for months following birth, which is a significant public health hazard because the virus can be transmitted to pregnant women. Some congenital shedders are asymptomatic and without malformations.
- Rubella virus **can be grown in cell culture.** It is identified in culture by its **ability to interfere with the CPE caused by ECHO virus.**
- Can also be diagnosed by serology in **hemagglutination inhibition test** or ELISA (four-fold rise in titer or presence of IgM antibody).
- IgM antibody indicates recent infection, whereas a 1:8 or greater titer of IgG antibody indicates immunity and thus protection.
- If recent infection has occurred, amniocentesis can reveal if there is rubella virus in the amniotic fluid, which indicates definite fetal infection.
- Prevention by **live attenuated vaccine** is effective and long lasting (at least 10 years); given

subcutaneously to children at 15 months of age in combination with measles and mumps vaccine, and to unimmunized young women if they are not pregnant and will use contraception for the next three months.

- As this is a live vaccine, should not be given to immunocompromised people or pregnant women

> **Confusing names:**
> Rubivirus—Rubella belongs to rubivirus group of Togaviridae
> Rubella—German measles
> Rubula—Mumps
> Rubeola—Measles

Other Togaviruses are described with Arboviruses

## RHABDOVIRUSES

### Rabies virus

- Single-stranded RNA virus, **bullet-shaped**, enveloped, negative polarity, so has RNA dependent RNA polymerase.
- **Single antigen type;** broad host range, can infect all mammals.
- Rabies virus attaches to acetylcholine receptor on the cell surface.
- Transmitted by the bite of rabid animal; could be dogs, cats or wild animals like bats, skunks.
- Rodents and rabbit do not transmit rabbits.
- **"Nonbite" exposures** can also result in rabies, e.g. exposure to aerosols of bat secretions.
- The virus multiplies locally at bite site, infects sensory neurons; and moves by axonal transport to central nervous system. Virus multiplies in the CNS and then travels down the peripheral nerves to the salivary glands and other organs. From the salivary glands, it enters the saliva to be transmitted by the bite. There is **no viremic stage.**
- Within CNS, encephalitis develops. Infected neurons contain an eosinophilic cytoplasmic

inclusion called **Negri Body**, which is important in laboratory diagnosis.

- Incubation varies from 2 to 16 weeks or more depending on the location of the bite.
- With progression of disease, **hydrophobia** develops, aversion to swallow water because of painful spasm of the throat.
- Disease is almost always fatal (few individuals have survived with the advent of life support systems).
- Rapid diagnosis in the animal is made by examination of brain tissue by using **fluorescent antibody** to rabies virus or histologic staining of Negri bodies in the cytoplasm of hippocampal neurons.
- Rabies in humans can be **diagnosed by fluorescent antibody staining** of biopsy specimen, usually taken from **skin of the neck at the hairline;** by isolation of virus from saliva, spinal fluid, and brain tissue; or by a rise in titer of antibody to the virus.
- Negri bodies can be demonstrated in **corneal scrapings** and in autopsy specimens of the brain.
- No antiviral therapy for patient with rabies.
- Prevention can be:
  - **Pre-exposure:** given to individuals in high-risk groups, such as veterinarian, zookeepers. Three doses on days 0, 7, and 21 or 28
  - **Postexposure:** routinely used after bite.
- Vaccine is an **inactivated virus grown in human diploid cells.** Duck embryo vaccine and nerve tissue vaccine are also available but not preferred.
- Postexposure immunization involves use of both vaccine and human rabies immune globulin (RIG) (obtained from hyperimmunized persons) plus immediate cleaning of the wound.
- Postexposure immunization depends on:
  - Type of animal
  - Whether animal was immunized or not
  - Wild or domestic animal

- Provoked or unprovoked attack
- Whether animal is available to be observed
- Whether rabies is endemic in that area.

- Five doses of HDCV are given (on days 0, 3, 7, 14, and 28), but RIG is given only once with the first dose of HDCV (at a different site to prevent neutralization).
- As much as possible RIG is given at the bite site, remaining given intramuscularly.
- If the animal has been captured, it should be **observed for 10 days.**
- Vaccine for immunization of animals (dogs) consists of inactivated rabies virus. First dose is given at 3 months of age, with booster doses given either annually or at 3 year intervals.

## RETROVIRUSES

- There are two important human retroviruses: Human T cell lymphotropic virus-1 (HTLV) and human immunodeficiency virus (HIV).
  - (HIV is described separately).
- Enveloped viruses with **reverse transcriptase;** two copies of a single stranded, positive polarity RNA genome.
- HTLV does not kill T cells, whereas HIV does.

## HTLV

- HTLV-1 causes:
  - a cancer called adult T cell leukemia/lymphoma (ATL) and
  - a neurologic disease called HTLV-associated myelopathy (HAM) (also known as tropical spastic paraparesis or chronic progressive myelopathy.
- Transmitted primarily by intravenous drug use, sexual contact, or breastfeeding.
- **Whole blood** and not plasma is a major source of transmission.
- ATL is characterized by lymphadenopathy, hepatosplenomegaly, lytic bone lesions, and skin

lesions. Blood shows malignant T cells that have a distinct flower-shaped nucleus.

- HAM shows gait disturbances, weakness of lower limbs. Loss of motor function is more than loss of sensory loss. T cells with a **'flower-shaped' nucleus** can be found in spinal fluid.
- Diagnosed by antibody detection using ELISA test, confirmed by Western Blot; PCR can also be done.

## RNA NONENVELOPED VIRUSES

## PICORNAVIRUSES

Small nonenveloped viruses, icosahedral, single stranded RNA, positive polarity.

**Two groups**:

*Enteroviruses:* include poliovirus, coxsackieviruses, echoviruses, Hepatitis A.

*Rhinoviruses:* Enteroviruses infect primarily the enteric tract, whereas rhinoviruses are found in the nose and throat.

### Enteroviruses

**Poliovirus**

- Causes poliomyelitis.
- Three serologic (antigenic) types.
- Transmitted by **fecal-oral route.**
- Polio eradication campaigns have led to elimination of polio from most parts of the world. India is close to achieving elimination. In 2005, till the writing of this book there were 14 cases, lowest ever and aim is to achieve zero wild transmission by the end of 2005.
- Vaccine used is live oral polio vaccine (**Sabin** vaccine) as it also provides herd immunity. Places where natural transmission has been stopped, killed vaccine **(Salk)** vaccine is used. Live vaccine should not be given to immunocompromised individuals.
- Poliovirus preferentially replicates in the motor neurons located in the anterior horn of the spinal

cord. Death of the cells results in **flaccid paralysis** of the muscles innervated by those neurons.

- Asymptomatic infection is quite common. Roughly 1% infections are clinically apparent.
- Poliovirus infection may range from:
  1. In apparent asymptomatic infection
  2. Abortive poliomyelitis—most common
  3. Nonparalytic poliomyelitis—presents as aseptic meningitis
  4. Paralytic poliomyelitis—flaccid paralysis, can also lead to respiratory paralysis.
- Diagnosis made either by isolation of the virus or by rise in antibody titer. Virus can be recovered from the throat, stool, or spinal fluid by inoculation in cell cultures.

**Coxsackie viruses**

- **Group A** cause herpangina, **acute hemorrhagic conjunctivitis** (especially Coxsackie A24), and hand-foot and mouth disease
- **Group B** cause pleurodynia (**Bornholm disease**, 'devil's grip'), **myocarditis**, and pericarditis; also associated with juvenile diabetes especially type B4
- Both types cause common cold and aseptic meningitis
- Diagnosis and group classification is based on pathogenicity in **suckling mice**
  - Group A causes widespread myositis and flaccid paralysis, which is rapidly fatal
  - Group B causes generalized less severe lesions of the heart, pancreas, CNS and local myositis
- Group A has 24 serotypes while Group B has 6

**ECHO viruses**

- ***E****nteric* ***C****ytopathogenic* ***H****uman* ***O****rphan viruses.* Although called 'orphan' because they were not initially associated with any disease, they are now known to cause variety of diseases like aseptic meningitis, respiratory infections, infantile diarrhea, hemorrhagic conjunctivitis.

- Along with coxsackie viruses these are **leading causes of aseptic (viral) meningitis**

**Other Enteroviruses**

**Enterovirus 70**: Main cause of acute hemorrhagic conjunctivitis

**Enterovirus 71**: Important cause of CNS infections, including meningitis, encephalitis, and paralysis.

**Enterovirus 72**: Hepatitis A virus. Described in detail with hepatitis viruses.

**Rhinoviruses**

- **Main cause of common cold.**
- More than 100 serologic types.
- Replicate better at 33°C than at 37°C, which explains why they affect primarily the nose and conjunctive rather than lower respiratory tract.
- They are acid labile, so do not cause gastrointestinal infections.
- Transmitted either from person to person via aerosols of respiratory droplets or indirectly through droplets deposited on hands or surfaces and transmitted by fingers to nose or eyes.

## CALICIVIRUSES

Small, nonenveloped viruses, single-stranded RNA with positive polarity.

Important pathogens include:

- **Hepatitis E:** described with other hepatitis viruses.
- **Norwalk virus.**

**Norwalk virus (Norovirus)**

- Common cause of viral gastroenteritis in adults.
- Transmitted by feco-oral route, commonly with contaminated seafood and water.
- Resistant to inactivation by chlorination and drying.
- **Watery diarrhea** with sudden onset vomiting.

**Reoviruses**

REO is an acronym for Respiratory, Enteric, Orphan

Rota virus is the most important member.

**Rotavirus**

- It is the **most common cause** of diarrhea in young children.
- **Segmented, double-stranded RNA virus.**
- Virus is released from the cytoplasm by lysis and not by budding.
- Transmitted by feco-oral route.
- **Watery diarrhea** caused by stimulation of enteric nervous system.
- Characterized by watery, non-bloody diarrhea, vomiting; most serious in young children.
- Diagnosis can be made by **detection of rotavirus in stool**.
- A **Rhesus reassortment vaccine** (tetravalent) was used in western countries till recent past but due to increased incidence of intussusceptions, went into disrepute and was discontinued.
- Live attenuated rotavirus vaccine is under trial in India currently.

## HEPATITIS VIRUSES

Known as hepatitis viruses because these are primarily hepatotropic (infect liver).

### Hepatitis A Virus

- Enterovirus classified in picornavirus family.
- Single-stranded, nonenveloped, icosahedral symmetry.
- Also known as **enterovirus 72**, hepatovirus, heparnavirus.
- Has one serotype.
- Transmitted by **fecal-oral route**; virus appears in stools two weeks before appearance of symptoms. Rarely transmitted by blood.
- Children are most frequently infected.

- Incubation period is 3-4 weeks as compared to Hepatitis B, which is 10-12 weeks.
- Most cases resolve spontaneously in 2-4 weeks.
- **No chronic hepatitis** or chronic carrier state occurs, and there is no predisposition to cirrhosis or hepatocellular carcinoma.
- **Detection of IgM antibody** is most important for diagnosis.
- Active immunization with **vaccine** containing **inactivated HAV** is available. Two doses at an interval of 6-12 months are given. No subsequent booster is recommended.
- Vaccine is recommended for travelers to endemic countries, children and homosexual men.
- Proper hygiene is of prime importance.

### Hepatitis B Virus

- Member of Hepadnavirus family; causes Hepatitis B.
- It is 42 nm-enveloped virus (known as **Dane particle**), icosahedral, partially double-stranded circular DNA virus.
- Envelope contains a protein called surface antigen (HBsAg) (also known as **Australia antigen**), which is important for laboratory diagnosis and immunization.
- Contains a **DNA-dependent DNA polymerase** which has a reverse transcriptase activity as well.
- Electron microscopy shows 42 nm virions, and many 22 nm spheres and long filaments 22 nm wide, which are composed of surface antigen.
- In addition to HBsAg, there are two important antigens; the core antigen **(HBcAg)** and the **e** antigen **(HBeAg).**
- HBeAg is an important **indicator of transmissibility** because the e antigen is located on the core protein, which means the infectious particle must be present in the patient's blood.
- Humans are the only natural hosts of HBV. There is **no animal reservoir.**

- Modes of transmission are blood, sexual, and perinatal (from mother to newborn).
- About 5% of patients become **chronic carriers;** HbsAg persisting in blood for more than 6 months.
- High rate of **hepatocellular carcinoma** occurs in chronic carriers. Carcinogenesis is a result of **insertional mutagenesis.** Integration of HBV DNA could activate a cellular oncogene, leading to a loss of growth control.
- Chronic carriage is more likely when infection occurs in a newborn (90%) than in an adult.
- Lifelong immunity occurs after natural infection; **antibody against HBsAg is protective.**
- Some chronic carriers can have **chronic active hepatitis,** which can lead to cirrhosis and death.
- **HBsAg indicates HBV infection;** it appears during the incubation period and is detectable in most patients during the prodrome and acute disease. It falls to undetectable levels during convalescence in most case; prolonged presence (more than 6 months) indicates carrier state and the risk of chronic hepatitis and hepatic carcinoma; antibodies to surface antigen (anti-HBs Ab) are not detectable in acute disease or in chronic carrier state.
- There is a period of several weeks when HBsAg has disappeared and anti-HBs Ab is not yet detectable. This is the window period. At this time, anti- HBc Ab is positive and can be used to make diagnosis. IgM form of anti-HBc Ab is present during acute infection and disappears around 6 months after infection.
- HBeAg arises during incubation period and is present during the prodrome and early acute disease and in certain chronic carriers. Finding of HBeAg indicates transmissibility and finding of antibodies (anti-HBeAb) indicates low transmissibility.
- HBV DNA in the serum is strong evidence that infectious virions are present.

- Alpha interferon is clinically useful for treatment of chronic hepatitis B infections; Lamivudine, adefovir are also useful.
- Prevention involves use of either the vaccine or hyperimmune globulin or both.
- The **vaccine contains HBsAg** produces in yeasts by **recombinant DNA techniques.**
- Hepatitis B immune globulin are given for passive protection to individuals exposed to HBsAg positive blood, e.g. after needle stick injury.
- All blood for transfusion should be screened for HBsAg; no one with history of hepatitis should donate blood.

| *Serological marker* | *Acute disease* | *Window Period* | *Complete recovery* | *Chronic carrier* | *Vaccinated* |
|---|---|---|---|---|---|
| HBsAg | Positive | Negative | Negative | Positive | Negative |
| Anti-HBs Ab | Negative | Negative | Positive | Negative | Positive |
| Anti- HBc Ab | Positive (IgM in acute stage, IgG in subsequent stages) | Positive | Positive | Positive | Negative |

## Hepatitis C virus

- Member of Hepacivirus group of flavivirus family; causes hepatitis C.
- Enveloped, single-stranded, positive polarity RNA.
- HCV has at least 6 genotypes.
- Genetic variability is due to high mutation rate in the envelope gene coupled with absence of a proofreading function in the RNA polymerase. As a result, multiple subspecies (quasi species) often occur in the blood of an infected individual at the same time.
- Transmitted primarily through blood.
- Unlike other flaviviruses, there is no evidence of an insect vector for HCV.
- HCV infection strongly predisposes to **hepatocellular carcinoma**; the mechanism is different from Hepatitis B virus. In HCV, it is an indirect mechanism as a result of metabolic derangement, while in Hepatitis B it is direct oncogenicity.

- Alcoholism enhances rate of hepatocellular carcinoma in HCV infected individuals.
- Approximately **75% of patients are chronically infected** and continue to produce virus for more than 1 year; rate of chronic carriage is much higher than HBV. Chronic active hepatitis and cirrhosis occurs in approximately 10% of these patients.
- Mean incubation period is 8 weeks.
- Cirrhosis resulting form HCV is a common indication for liver transplantation.
- HCV infection also **leads to significant autoimmune reactions,** including vasculitis, purpura, arthralgias and membranoproliferative glomerulonephritis.
- HCV is the main cause of **essential mixed cryoglobulinemia.**
- HCV infection is diagnosed by detecting antibodies to HCV by ELISA. The test does not distinguish between acute, chronic or resolved infection. Because false positive results can occur in ELISA, **an RIBA (recombinant immunoblot assay)** should be performed as a confirmatory test. PCR based test should be performed in RIBA positive cases to determine if active disease exists.
- Chronic infection is characterized by detectable viral RNA for at least 6 months.
- Treatment with **alpha interferon** significantly decreases number of patients that become chronic carriers; combination of alpha interferon and ribavirin is treatment of choice for chronic hepatitis C.

**Hepatitis D Virus (Delta virus)**

- Unusual in that it is a **defective virus;** it cannot replicate by itself but only in cells also infected with Hepatitis B virus. HBV is, therefore, a helper virus for HDV.
- HDV is enveloped RNA virus with single-stranded, negative polarity, covalently closed circle.
- HDV replicates in the nucleus.

- Transmitted by blood, sexually or perinatally.
- HDV could coinfect or superinfect patients with HBV; **superinfection is much more severe** and the incidence of fulminant, life-threatening hepatitis, chronic hepatitis, and liver failure is significantly higher.
- Diagnosis made by detecting delta antigen or IgM antibody to delta antigen in patient's serum.

### Hepatitis E Virus

- Tentatively a member of family Calicivirus.
- Nonenveloped, icosahedral, positive polarity, single stranded RNA virus.
- Transmitted by **fecal-oral route**; usually contaminated drinking water source.
- Generally occurs in **'e'pidemics;** infective dose is high (unlike hepatitis A, which requires low infective dose and occurs sporadically throughout the year as a result of direct contact with contaminated material).
- Resolves spontaneously in most people, but causes severe, **life-threatening fulminant hepatitis in pregnant women.** The reason for this predisposition is not clear.
- Does not causes chronicity, cirrhosis or carcinoma.
- India is endemic for Hepatitis E.
- Delhi and Kashmir had large outbreaks of hepatitis E in past. These were labeled as non-A non-B hepatitis till hepatitis E was discovered. Sera from those unidentified outbreaks revealed Hepatitis E. Such technique is known as **'seroarchaeology'**.
- HEV infection is diagnosed by ruling out other common causes like HAV.
- **Immune electron microscopy (IEM)** can demonstrate HEV in stool.

### Hepatitis G Virus

- Also known as GB virus type C.
- Belongs to same group as Hepatitis C virus, i.e. Hepacivirus group of **Flaviviridae family.**

- Enveloped, single-stranded, positive polarity RNA
- Transmitted by **parenteral route,** i.e. blood and sexual.
- It is not clear whether HGV causes hepatitis on its own or exacerbated disease caused by other hepatitis viruses.
- Strangely **coinfection of HIV and HGV leads to lower mortality** as compared to individuals infected with HIV alone.

### Transfusion Transmitted Virus (TTV)

- Member of Circoviridae, a plant virus group, which has single-stranded DNA.
- Shown in post-transfusion hepatitis but association not clear yet.

## ARBOVIRUSES

Arthropod borne viruses, i.e. transmitted by arthropods, like mosquitoes and ticks. It is not a taxonomic term but a collective name for a large group of diverse viruses. Diseases caused are mainly, **viral encephalitis** or **viral hemorrhagic fevers.**

Most arboviruses belong to:

- **Togaviruses:** Icosahedral, enveloped, single stranded, positive polarity RNA virus; two groups: **alphaviruses** and rubivirus. Rubivirus has rubella described separately. Alphaviruses are arboviruses, e.g. eastern equine encephalitis, western equine encephalitis, Chikungunya, O' Nyong Nyong, Ross River, Semliki Forest Virus.
- **Flaviviruses:** Isosahedral, enveloped, single stranded, positive polarity RNA, e.g. Mosquito borne like St Louis encephalitis, yellow fever, dengue fever, West Nile virus, Japanese encephalitis, or tick borne like Kyasanur Forest Disease in Mysore. (Hepatitis C and G viruses also belong to flaviviruses but are not arboviruses).
- **Bunyaviruses:** Helical, enveloped, segmented, negative sense RNA virus, e.g. Mosquito borne

like Bunyamwera, Oropuche, Tick borne like Crimean Congo hemorrhagic fever, Bhanja virus.

## ROBOVIRUSES

Viruses transmitted by rodents:

- **Arenaviruses**: Isosahedral, enveloped, segmented, ambisense RNA virus also known as **"sandy viruses"** generally cause hemorrhagic fevers, e.g. New world viruses like Junin, Machupo, Guanarito, or Old World viruses like Lassa fever, Lymphocytic choriomeningitis virus (LCM)
- **Hantaviruses**: Members of bunyaviruses. All bunyaviruses are arboviruses except hantaviruses which are roboviruses (rodent borne). Hantaviruses cause **Hemorrhagic fever renal syndrome (HFRS),** e.g. Hantaan virus, Thottapalayam, or **Hantavirus Pulmonary syndrome** e.g. Sin Nombre.

## FILOVIRUSES

### Ebola and Marburg viruses

- Members of Filoviruses, which are filamentous viruses.
- Ebola has four types: Zaire, Sudan, Reston and Ivory Coast.
- Ebola-Zaire is the most virulent; Cause hemorrhagic fever with almost 100% mortality.
- Marburg has one serotype; it is associated with lowest mortality rates.

### Borna Disease Virus

- Helical, negative sense, single-stranded, non-segmented RNA virus.
- Has been associated with **psychiatric illnesses** like bipolar mood disorders and schizophrenia.

## HUMAN IMMUNODEFICIENCY VIRUS (HIV)

Causes acquired immunodeficiency syndrome (AIDS).

### Important Properties

- Two types: HIV-1 and HIV-2; **HIV-1** is more common worldwide
- HIV preferentially infects and kills helper **(CD4)** T lymphocytes, resulting in loss of cell-mediated immunity and a high probability of opportunistic infections. Other cells like macrophages and monocytes are also infected especially in the early part of infection in a new host
- HIV belongs to lentivirus subgroup of retroviruses.
- Two identical molecules of single-stranded, positive polarity RNA; said to be diploid
- In addition to three typical retroviral genes ***gag***, ***pol*** and ***env***, which code for structural proteins, also has six regulatory genes, ***tat*** (transactivator of transcription) and **rev** required for replication and other four ***nef*** (negative factor), ***vif*** (viral infectivity factor), ***vpu*** and ***vpr***, are termed as accessory genes.
- The '***gag***' gene codes for internal '**core**' proteins, most important of which is **p24**, an antigen used in serologic tests.
- The '***pol***' gene encodes for several proteins including '**reverse transcriptase**' (RNA-dependent DNA-polymerase), which synthesizes DNA by using RNA as a template, an **integrase** that integrates the viral DNA into the cellular DNA, and a **protease** that cleaves the various viral precursor proteins.
- The '***env***' gene codes for gp 160, a precursor glycoprotein that is cleaved to form the two envelope (surface) glycoproteins, **gp 120 and gp 41.**
- HIV-1 is divided into groups M (major), N and O (outliers); M is the most common.
- On the basis of gene that codes for gp120, HIV is divided into subtypes (clades) A through I.
- **Clade C** is the commonest in India (C3 being the commonest subtype); Clade A and B are also found in India.

- The subtypes are differentiated using **heteroduplex mobility assay (HMA)**
- Important antigens of HIV:
  - gp 120 and gp 41 are the type specific envelope glycoproteins. gp 120 protrudes from the surface and interacts with the CD4 receptor on the cell surface (and a second chemokine receptor, CCR5. People with mutated CCR5 receptor are resistant to HIV infection). The gene that codes for gp 120 mutates rapidly, resulting in many antigenic variants. Antibodies against gp 120 neutralize the infectivity of HIV but the rapid appearance of gp 120 variants will make production of an effective vaccine difficult. The high mutation rate may be due to lack of editing (splicing) function in the reverse transcriptase
  - p 24 is the group specific antigen, located in the core and not known to vary.
- Humans are the natural hosts although some primates can be infected in the laboratory
- There is evidence that chimpanzees in West Africa were the source of HIV-1.

## Transmission and Epidemiology

- Transmission of HIV occurs primarily by **sexual contact** and by **transfer of infected blood. Perinatal transmission** from infected mother to neonate also occurs either across the **placenta, at birth, or via breast milk.** It is estimated that more than 50% neonatal infections occur at the time of delivery, and roughly half of remaining are either through placenta or through breastfeeding.
- HIV is transmitted less effectively as compared to Hepatitis B.
- Also found in other fluids like saliva and tears, but role in infection is not clear.
- People with other STD especially with ulcerative lesions have a significantly higher risk of transmitting and acquiring HIV.

- First reported in 1981, worldwide there are estimated 40 million people infected, two-thirds of whom are in sub-Saharan Africa.
- Now **fourth leading cause of death worldwide;** after ischemic heart disease, cerebrovascular disease, and acute lower respiratory infections.
- **India has 5.1 million HIV infected individuals**
- Risk of being infected after **percutaneous** exposure to HIV-infected blood is estimated to be about **0.3%.**
- Antibodies to HIV typically appear 3-4 weeks after infection; HIV can be transmitted to others during this period
- The late stage of HIV infection is AIDS, manifested by a decline in the number of CD4 cells to below 400/μl and an increase in the frequency and severity of opportunistic infections

### Clinical Findings

- Most characteristic manifestations are Pneumocystis pneumonia and Kaposi's sarcoma.
- Other opportunistic infections include bacterial infections like disseminated **Mycobacterium tuberculosis** and **Mycobacterium avium intercellulare** infections, fungal infections such as thrush (caused by **Candida albicans**), cryptococcal meningitis, disseminated histoplasmosis, protozoal infections like toxoplamosis and cryptosporidiosis, viral infections like disseminated herpes simplex, herpes zoster, cytomegalovirus and progressive multifocal leucoencephalopathy.

### Laboratory Diagnosis

- Presumptive diagnosis is made by detection of antibodies by ELISA, but as there could be false positive results confirmation in made by Western blot analysis
- For routine diagnosis in developing country settings **ERS (ELISA, Rapid, Simple) strategies** are used, i.e. instead of Western Blot series of

serological tests are carried out depending on the situation:

- **ERS-1** strategy is used for blood banks; positive test is an indication for discarding the blood bag
- **ERS-2** strategy is used for volunteers or donors
- **ERS-3** strategy is used for suspected cases; people presenting with features of infections or AIDS defining illnesses.

- PCR is a very sensitive and specific that can be used to detect HIV in infected cells. The viral load can also be determined by PCR, which defines the **prognosis and response to therapy.**
- During first month of infection, diagnosis of acute HIV infection can be made by either viral culture, p24 antigen test or PCR assay. Increase in HIV RNA can be detected by PCR in 10-20 days while p24 antigen increase can be seen in 30 days in patients whose antibody tests are negative.

### Treatment

- Current regimen consists of two **nucleoside inhibitors** (zidovudine and lamivudine) and a **protease inhibitor** (indinavir). This combination is known as **HAART (highly active anti-retroviral therapy).** It is effective in prolonging life, improving quality of life and reducing viral load but does not cure chronic HIV infection, i.e. latent infection of CD-4 positive cells continues indefinitely. Other drugs are also used in various combinations including **non-nucleoside reverse transcriptase inhibitor**, efavirenz; Didanosine, zalcitabine, stavudine, Nevirapine, delavirdine, saquinavir, ritonavir, are other choices. A new class of drug known as **fusion inhibitors**, enfuvirtide, has also been approved recently.
- Prevention consists of measures to avoid exposure to the virus, e.g. using condoms, not sharing needles and discarding donated blood that is contaminated with HIV.

- **ABC** of HIV prevention are **Abstinence, Be faithful** to partner and use **Condoms.**
- Postexposure prophylaxis, such as given after needle stick injury, consists of zidovudine, lamivudine and indinavir.
- Perinatal infections in children can be reduced by.
- AZT or nevirapine should be given perinatally to HIV infected mother and neonate, and HIV infected mother should not breastfeed. In addition, delivery should be accomplished by cesarean section rather than vaginal delivery.
- Several drugs are required to prevent and treat certain opportunistic infections.

## PRIONS

- Prions are **proteinecous infectious particles** that have no detectable nucleic acid.
- These are highly resistant to inactivation by heat, formaldehyde, and proteases.
- Normal cellular prior protein $PrP^{c}$ with alpha helical structure may change to abnormal $PrP^{sc}$ due to conformational change to beta plated sheets. Prions replicate by abnormal forms recruiting normal forms and changing their conformation to make them abnormal.
- Human prion-mediated disease, e.g. kuru and Creutzfeldt Jacob disease (CJD) are called **transmissible spongiform encephalopathies.** The term spongiform refers to the spongy, Swiss cheese like holes seen in brain parenchyma that are caused by death of the neurons.
- Kuru, variant CJD and bovine spongiform encephalopathy (or **mad cow disease**) can be acquired by ingestion .
- Prion diseases can be classified into three types:
  - Transmissible (infectious) such as kuru
  - Hereditary (genetic) such as fatal familial insomnia
  - Sporadic (neither infectious nor genetic) such as most cases of CJD due to spontaneous somatic mutations.

- There are cases of CJD that are due to mutation in germ cells and others transmitted either iatrogenically via brain electrodes and growth hormones or by eating contaminated beef.

Features of human prion diseases

| *Disease* | *Pathogenesis* | *Important feature* |
|---|---|---|
| Kuru | Transmissible/ infectious | Caused by ingesting or handling brain tissue. Occurred in Papua New Guinea tribes people, who practiced cannibalism |
| Creutzfeldt-Jacob disease | 1. Transmissible/ infectious | Iatrogenic transmission by corneal transplant, brain electrode, and growth hormone |
| | 2. Hereditary/ genetic | Mutation in germ cells |
| | 3. Sporadic | No relationship to any known cause; possible new mutation in somatic cells; most common form |
| Variant Creutzfeldt Jacob disease | Transmissible/ infectious | Probably acquired by eating meat or nervous tissue from animals with 'mad cow' disease |
| Gerstmann-Staussler-Scheinker syndrome | Hereditary/ genetic | Mutation in germ cells |
| Fatal familial insomnia | Hereditary/ genetic | Mutation in germ cells |

**Prion diseases of animals:**

**Scrapie** is a disease of sheep

**Bovine spongiform encephalopathy (BSE)**: also known as **mad cow disease**. Normally prions do not jump species barrier, but in case of BSE, transmission from sheep to cattle took place thus raising concern of further transmission to human beings. The prions isolated from variant CJD cases in humans have found to resemble the prions isolated from mad cow disease, which is evidence to support the hypothesis that variant CJD originated by eating beef.

**Chronic wasting disease:** prion disease of deer and elk.

CHAPTER SEVEN

# High Frequency Points

## GENERAL MICROBIOLOGY

### STRUCTURE AND FUNCTION

- Prokaryotes (bacteria) **lack nucleus**, nuclear membrane and organelles like mitochondria and Golgi bodies.
- Prokaryotes have **cell wall** (which is unique to them as eukaryotes lack cell wall).
- Based on cell wall structure: **Gram-positive** and **gram-negative** bacteria.
- Gram-negative cell wall has **Lipopolysaccharide (LPS)**, which functions as **endotoxin.** Therefore only gram-negative organisms can form endotoxin.
- Gram-positive cell wall has **teichoic acids**.
- Both gram-positive and gram-negative organisms can produce exotoxins.
- Maximum exotoxin production is seen in **log (exponential) phase** of bacterial growth curve.
- Flagella are organs of locomotion (**motility**) in bacteria:
  - Monotrichous—*Vibrio cholerae*- **darting** motility
  - Amphitrichous—*Listeria*- **tumbling** motility
  - Lophotrichous—*Helicobacter*.
  - Peritrichous—Motile members of *Enterobacteriaceae* family e.g. *E. coli*, *Salmonella*, *Proteus*, which show **stately** motility.
  - Endoflagellum: Spirochaetes: **corkscrew** motility.

- **Twitching** motility in *Eikenella* is because of pili.

• Pili (fimbriae) are means of **adhesion.**

• Bacterial **genetics.**
  - Specialized pili (sex pili) carry out **conjugation** (transfer of genetic material from one bacterium to another
  - **Transformation**: acquisition of new genetic material through naked DNA demonstrated in pneumococci by Griffith experiment
  - **Transduction**: transfer of genetic material into bacteria by bacteriophage (virus)
  - **Transposon**: jumping genes—discovered by Barbara McClintok- Nobel prize.

• **Staining** methods:
  - Gram staining: differential staining
  - Ziehl-Neelsen staining: acid-fast staining- Mycobacteria, nocardia, etc.
  - Kinyoun staining: cold acid-fast staining: *Cryptosporidium parvum*
  - Albert staining: metachromatic staining- *Corynebacterium diphtheriae*
  - Giemsa, Leishman, Wright, Field, JSB stains: Romanowsky stains.

• **Growth** Requirements:
  - Obligate Aerobes: grow only in presence of oxygen, e.g. *Bacillus*
  - Facultative Anaerobes: grow better in presence but can grow in absence of oxygen as well, e.g. *Enterobacteriaceae* family
  - Obligate Anaerobes: grow only in absence of oxygen e.g. *Clostridium*
  - Microaerophilic: grow best in 3-5% oxygen, e.g. *Helicobacter*
  - Capnophilic: grow well with additional 5-10% carbon dioxide, e.g. pneumococci, meningococci, *H. influenzae*.

• **Culture** media:
  - Transport media: Cary Blair medium (universal transport medium)

VR fluid—*Vibrio cholerae*
Stuart's transport medium: respiratory specimen
- Enrichment media: Selenite F broth-*Salmonella, Shigella.*
  VR fluid, Alkaline peptone water- *Vibrio cholerae*.
- Enriched media: Blood Agar, Chocolate agar
- Selective media: Wilson Blair medium: Salmonella.
  Potassium tellurite blood agar: *Corynebacterium diphtheriae.*
- Medium for Mycobacteria: Lowenstein Jensen medium, Middlebrook medium.
- Medium for Corynebacterium: Loeffler's serum slope.

• Antibiotic susceptibility testing done by diffusion methods or dilution methods.
• Disc diffusion methods: Stokes method, Kirby Bauer method.
• Dilution methods: for calculating **minimum inhibitory concentration.**
• **Serological tests:**
  - Slide agglutination—blood grouping, serotyping of *Salmonella*
  - Tube agglutination—Widal test
  - Slide flocculation—VDRL
  - Tube flocculation—Kahn test
  - Complement fixation test—Wasserman test.
• **Molecular** tests
  - **Polymerase chain reaction**: amplification method, done in thermocycler, Steps-denaturation (94-96°C), annealing (54°C) and extension (72°C). Enzyme used Taq polymerase. Gel stained by ethidium bromide.
    - Multiplex PCR: diagnosing many organisms in one PCR, e.g. CSF sample
    - Nested PCR: increases specificity
    - Reverse Transcriptase **(RT)-PCR**: quantitation

- Arbitrarily primed PCR (**AP-PCR**) or Randomly Amplified Polymorphic DNA (RAPD)—used for epidemiological typing or strain differentiation
- Ligase chain reaction (**LCR**): amplification method, does not require thermocycler
- **b-DNA**: quantitation method without thermocycler
- Pulsed Field gel electrophoresis (**PFGE**): best method (gold standard) of epidemiological typing.

- **Sterilization and disinfection**
  - **Hot air oven**: 160°C for 1 hour. Glassware, oils, wax, powders, sharp instruments.
  - **Autoclaving:** 121°C for 15-20 minutes at 15 pounds per square inch pressure. Gloves, masks, gowns, linen, cotton, rubber plastic containing articles, surgical instruments, catheters, agar.
  - **Inspissation:** not a method of sterilization. Only a method of solidifying media containing serum (LSS) or egg (LJ) (80°C for 30 minutes).
  - **Tyndallization**: method of sterilization for media containing egg or serum. (80°C for 30 minutes for three consecutive days with intermittent overnight incubation at 37°C).
  - **Filteration**: for heat sensitive fluids. Vaccines, antibiotic solutions, serum, sugar containing media.
  - Low temperature steam formaldehyde **(LTSF), Gas Plasma**: newer methods for heat sensitive articles.
  - **Bulk sterilization**: Gamma radiation or ethylene oxide.
  - **UV rays:** not able to sterilize, just surface disinfectants.
  - Chemical sterilization: **Glutaraldehyde** (2% Cidex) for endoscopes.
  - Universal disinfectant: **Hypochlorite** (bleaching agent).

- **Biological indicators** of sterilization: Bacterial spores (*Bacillus steareothermophilus*, *Clostridium tetani* var. *niger*).

## VIROLOGY

- Viruses classified on the basis of **type of nucleic acid**: DNA viruses and RNA viruses.
- Other features for classification: symmetry, envelope, number of strands.
- **Non-enveloped viruses** can infect through feco-oral route, enveloped viruses cannot..
- Viruses can be grown by: animal inoculation, egg inoculation and cell cultures.
- Parts of embryonated egg:
  - **Amniotic fluid**—for primary isolation
  - **Yolk sac**—vaccine production
  - **Allantoic cavity**—antigen production for diagnostic kits
  - **Chorioallantoic membrane (CAM)**—differentiation of pox viruses, herpes viruses
- Cell cultures: **Primary cell culture:** primary isolation

  **Semi-continuous or diploid culture**: vaccine production

  **Continuous cell lines** (derived from malignant cells): antigen production for diagnostic kits.
- All DNA viruses are double-stranded except Parvoviruses {and now Circoviridae (TTV) also}.
- All DNA virus families have oncogenic members except Parvoviridae.
- Parvovirus B 19 (**Erythrovirus B19**) causes **fifth disease**, also called erythema infectiosum, which gives a typical **slapped cheek appearance**, associated with hydrops fetalis and can cause aplastic crisis in sickle cell anemia.
- Papovaviridae now divided into two families: Papillomaviridae (which has Human Papilloma virus) and Polyomaviridae (which has JC virus, BK virus, SV 40).
- **JC virus** causes progressive multifocal leucoencephalopathy.

- Adenoviruses cause respiratory infections, hemorrhagic conjunctivitis, infantile gastroenteritis (**adeno type 40, 41**).
- Human herpes viruses:
  1. Herpes simplex virus 1 (**HSV-1**)—lesions above the waist.
  2. Herpes simplex virus 2 (**HSV-2**)—lesions below the waist and herpes encephalitis.
  3. Varicella zoster virus (**VZV**)—chickenpox and shingles.
  4. Ebstein barr virus (**EBV**)—infectious mononucleosis, Burkitt's lymphoma, nasopharyngeal carcinoma.
  5. Cytomegalovirus (**CMV**)—congenital infection, CMV inclusion disease (CID), CMV chorioretinitis (earliest sign of AIDS related illness).
  6. HHV 6- **roseola** virus, sixth disease.
  7. HHV 7.
  8. **Kaposi sarcoma related virus**: AIDS defining illness.
- Pox viruses are the largest viruses, some of them can be seen by a light microscope.
- Pox viruses are **brick-shaped.**
- All DNA viruses multiply in the nucleus except poxviruses, which multiply in the cytoplasm.
- Variola (smallpox), Vaccinia (vaccine strain), molluscum contagiosum, cowpox, buffalopox, avian-pox, monkeypox are Pox viruses but chickenpox virus is a Herpes virus.
- Molluscum contagiosum and Hepatitis B are examples of **non-cultivable** viruses.

### Hepatitis Viruses

Hepatitis A: RNA virus, Picornaviridae, feco-oral transmission, person to person transmission, no chronicity, no malignancy, no fulminancy, no cirrhosis

Hepatitis E: RNA virus, Caliciviridae, feco-oral transmission, causes outbreaks/epidemics, fulminant disease in pregnant females, no chronicity, no malignancy, no cirrhosis.

Hepatitis B: DNA virus, Hepadnaviridae, Partial double strand, serological markers:
HBsAg: denotes infection
HBeAg: denotes active multiplication, infectivity
(HbcAg: does not come in blood)
IgM Anti-HBc: depicts recent infection, best serological marker in window period
Anti-Hbe: recovering, good prognosis
Anti-HBs: immunized- recovered or vaccinated
HBV DNA: best marker in window period, response to therapy, prognosis

Hepatitis C: RNA virus, Flaviviridae, parenteral transmission, best marker for prognosis is viral load done by RT-PCR, 15% true responders to interferon therapy

Hepatitis D: deficient virus, superinfection with Hepatitis B more lethal than coinfection

Hepatitis G: RNA virus, Flaviviridae (same as Hepatitis C), also known as GBV-C

TTV: Transfusion transmitted virus, Circoviridae, single-stranded DNA virus

- **Picornaviridae**:
  - Polioviruses: Pulse polio immunization based on herd immunity
  - Oral polio vaccine: Live attenuated, Sabin vaccine
  - Killed Polio vaccine: Salk vaccine
  - Rhinoviruses: commonest cause of common cold
  - ECHO viruses: Enteric cytopathogenic human orphan virus
  - Coxsachie A & B
  - Type A 24 causes hemorrhagic conjunctivitis, and Type B causes myocarditis

  - Hepatovirus: Hepatitis A virus, earlier known as enterovirus type 72
  - Enterovirus type 68-71: Type 70 causes hemorrhagic conjunctivitis.
- **Astro** viruses–star-shaped viruses.
- **Reoviruses**: Double-stranded RNA viruses, Segmented.
  Most important member:
  Rotavirus: commonest cause of diarrhea in children below 5 years of age.
- Togaviridae: **Rubella**, which causes German measles (**Rubeola** is measles and **Rubula** is mumps).
- **Segmented viruses: B O A R.**
  Bunyaviridae, Orthomyxov., Arenav., Reov.
- **Arbo viruses**: arthropod borne viruses, not a taxonomic term, common diseases are hemorrhagic fevers, viral encephalitis, commonly members of Flaviviridae (e.g. Dengue, Yellow Fever, Japanese Encephalitis), Arenaviridae (e.g. Junin, Machupo, Guanarito, EEE, VEE), Bunyaviridae (e.g. Bunyamvera).
- Arenaviruses: sandy viruses, segmented, **ambi-sense.**
- Corona virus: respiratory viruses, most important member: **SARS** (Severe acute respiratory syndrome)—mutant Corona Virus.
- Retroviruses: only RNA viruses to multiply in the nucleus.
- All retroviruses are oncogenic except HIV.
- Commonest subtype in India **is HIV 1 subtype C3**, India also has subtypes A and B.
- **ERS: (ELISA, Rapid, Simple)** strategies are used for routine diagnosis.
  ERS 1: Blood banks
  ERS 2: Volunteers
  ERS 3: Symptomatic suspected cases
- RT PCR (viral load) is the best marker for prognosis

- **Negative sense RNA viruses:** Bunyaviridae, Orthomyxov., Paramyxov., Rhabdov., **Bornav.** {new family possibly associated with psychiatric (bipolar) disorders}, Filov.
- All bunyaviruses are arboviruses except Hantaviruses.
- **Hantaviruses** cause hemorrhagic fever renal syndrome and Hantavirus pulmonary syndrome.
- Othromyxoviruses: Influenza viruses show **antigenic shift** (results in pandemics) and **antigenic drift** (results in epidemics). **Avian influenza** (bird flu) virus is H5N1.
- Paramyxoviruses include measles, mumps and respiratory syncytial virus (RSV). **RSV** is the commonest cause of acute bronchiolitis in children.
- Rabies virus is rhabdovirus, it is a **bullet-shaped** virus.
- Rabies vaccine used in humans is human diploid cell vaccine.
- **Ebola virus** is a Filovirus. Most virulent is Ebola-Zaire variety.

## MYCOLOGY

- Fungi can be true yeasts, true hyphae or dimorphic (yeast at 37°C, hyphae at 22°C- thermal dimorphism).
- Fungi can multiply by sexual or asexual sporulation
- Fungi are classified on the basis of **sexual spores** into phylla:
  - Ascomycota (that form **ascospore**)
  - Basidiomycota (that form **basidiospore)**
  - Zygomycota (that form **zygospore).**
- Members of Ascomycota cause:superficial, subcutaneous and deep/systemic infections.
- **Superficial infections:** diagnosed by **10% KOH** preparation followed by culture on Sabaraoud's dextrose agar (SDA) and morphology of fungal growth on **LPCB** (Lacto Phenol Cotton Blue dye). **White piedra**: *Trichosporon* species.

**Black piedra**: *Piedraria hortae*
**Tinea nigra**: *Hortae* (formerly *Exophiala) werneckii*
**Dermatophytes:** (ringworm or Tinea infections: misnomer), asexual spores are called **conidia** or aleurispores, differentiation is done on the basis of morphology and distribution of micro- and macroconidia

- ***Trichophyton:*** causes infections of hair nail and skin, commonest species in *T. rubrum.*
  ***Microsporum:*** causes infections of hair and skin
- ***Epidermophyton***: causes infections of nail and skin
- **Subcutaneous infections**:
  ***Sporothrix schenckii***: causes sporotrichosis, **dimorphic** fungi causing subcutaneous mycoses, associated with vegetative matter injury like thorn prick or wooden splinters, therefore especially associated with farmers
- **Mycetoma:** Eumycetoma caused by fungi e.g. Madura foot caused by *Madurella madurai* (Actinomycotic mycetoma caused by bacteria). Diagnosed by KOH preparation and Gram staining of discharging granules.
- **Deep/ Systemic infections**:
  **Dimorphic fungi**:
  ***Histoplasma capsulatum***: transmitted by bats, differential diagnosis: LD bodies as macrophages are involved in both
  ***Blastomyces blastomyces***
  ***Coccidioides immitis***: spherules are seen
  ***Paracoccidioides braziliensis***: mickey mouse appearance, Mariner's wheel appearance
  ***Penicillium marneffii***: Corda's phenomenon seen, *P. marneffii* is one of the commonest opportunistic infections in HIV infected in South East Asia.
  ***Aspergillus***: hyaline fungus. *Aspergillus flavus*: Aflatoxin production—hepatotoxic.

*Aspergillus fumigatus*: Allergic broncho-pulmonary aspergillosis—precondition associated with asthma.

**Candida**: can cause superficial, subcutaneous and deep infections. Most important is *Candia albicans*. Differentiated from other *Candida* species by **germ tube, pseudohyphae** and **chlamydospore** formation.

- **Demetecious fungi:** Black moulds. Generally laboratory contaminants but can cause keratitis and otitis media, e.g. *Curvalaria, Alternaria.*
- **Phaeohyphomycosis:** caused by phaeoid (dark) fungi.
- **Hyalohyphomycosis**: caused by hyaline fungi.
- **Chromoblastomycosis**: subcutaneous infection caused by dark fungi typified by presence of **muriform cells** or **sclerotic bodies.**
- Members of Basidiomycota:

  ***Mallesezia furfur:*** causes Pitryasis versicolor, shows tissue dimorphism, typical grapes and bananas or spaghetti and meatball appearance, olive oil overlay over SDA for culture.

  ***Cryptococcus neoformans:*** two varieties: var. neoformans transmitted by pigeon droppings var. gatti found in bark of eucalyptus trees Common cause of meningitis in immunocompromised, capsulated organism, true yeast, multiply by budding (blastospore formation), India ink staining (negative staining), Meyer's mucicarmine staining (capsule appears pink) for diagnosis, selective media is niger seed or bird seed agar. Urease positive organism.

## BACTERIOLOGY

- Gram staining is **differential** staining.
- Divides bacteria into **gram-positive (cocci and bacilli)** and gram-negative **(cocci and bacilli).**

### Gram-positive Cocci

- Divided into catalase positive and catalase negative: **Catalase Positive** gram-positive cocci: **Staphylococci** and **Micrococci.**

Micrococci are normal skin commensals usually seen in groups of 4. (*M. agilis* is motile gram-positive coccus)

Staphylococci and micrococci are distinguished on the basis of sensitivity to **furazolidone** and **bacitracin**. Staphylococci are furazolidone sensitive and bacitracin resistant while micrococci are otherwise.

*Staphylococcus aureus* is confirmed by **coagulase** test. *S. aureus* shows β **hemolysis, golden yellow pigment** on blood agar. On Gram staining irregular grape like **clusters.**

*S. aureus* gastroenteritis is caused by preformed toxin, symptoms appear within 6 hours. Methicillin Resistant *Staphylococcus aureus* (**MRSA**) is a chromosomal resistance, mutation in mecA gene. Drug of choice for MRSA is Vancomycin. Carriage is maximum in external nares, carriers treated by mupirocin.

*Staph. epidermidis* is coagulase negative, associated with prosthetic valve and prosthetic joint infections.

*Staph saprophyticus* is novobiocin resistant, causes urinary tract infections.

**Catalase negative** gram-positive cocci: **Streptococci** and **Enterococci**

Streptococci are classified on the basis of carbohydrate C antigen in the cell wall. This is called **Lancefield grouping.**

Group A streptococci (*Strept. pyogenes*) are the most important in sore throat. Show β **hemolysis, pin point colonies** on blood agar. Associated with post-streptococcal glomerulonephritis and rheumatic fever. Group A is **bacitracin sensitive**.

Group B is **cAMP test** positive.

*Streptococcus pneumoniae* is capsulated, diplococcus, lanceolate-shaped, α hemolytic, **draughts-**

**man or carrom coin colonies**, optochin sensitive, show bile solubility and are **capnophilic** (grow well in 5-10% $CO_2$).

Enterococci can grow at 9.6 pH, 6.5% NaCl, 40% bile, and show bile esculin hydrolysis.

### Gram-positive Bacilli

**Obligate aerobes**

***Bacillus*:** Forms spores

*B. anthracis* causes anthrax, has polypeptide capsule, non-motile, shows **bamboo stick or boxcar** appearance, **inverted fir tree appearance** in gelatin stab, **Medusa Head** colonies.

*B. cereus* causes food poisoning associated with preformed toxin, symptoms appear within 12 hours, associated with **Chinese fried rice**.

*B. thuringensis* is used for biological control of vectors.

*B. steareothermophilus* is used as biological indicator of sterilization.

### Facultative Anaerobe

***Corynebacterium diphtheriae*** causes sore throat, diphtheria. No septicemia, only **toxemia**. Albert staining shows **metachromatic granules**, **Chinese letter** pattern, **cuneiform** arrangement. Cultured on **Loeffler's serum slope**, selective medium is **Potassium tellurite blood agar**.

### Obligate Anaerobe

***Clostridium*:** Forms spores

*C. perfringens* (previously *welchii*) causes gas gangrene

*C. tetani* causes tetanus

*C. difficile* associated with pseudomembranous (post-antibiotic) colitis

*C. botulinum* causes botulism. Botulinum toxin one of the most potent toxins

### Gram-negative Cocci

*Neisseria*: diplococci

*N. gonorrhoeae*: commonest cause of urethritis

*N. meningitidis* is capnophilic, causes meningitis.

### Gram-negative Bacilli

- Differentiated by oxidase test into oxidase negative and oxidase positive.

**Oxidase negative**: Family *Enterobacteriaceae*: members divided into lactose fermenting (pink colonies) and non-fermenting (colorless colonies).

**Lactose fermenting**:

Motile: *E. coli*

Nonmotile: *Klebsiella*

***E.coli***: Enterovirulent *E.coli*: EPEC associated with infantile diarrhea

ETEC causes traveler's diarrhea

EHEC associated with hemolytic uremic syndrome

*EIEC, EAEC, DAEC*

Uropathogenic *E.* coli possess p fimbriae

*E. coli* are used as markers of fecal contamination to assess bacteriological quality of water

***Klebsiella***: capsulated, mucoid colonies

**Non-lactose fermenting**: motile: *Salmonella, Proteus*

Nonmotile: *Shigella*

***Salmonella***: Cause enteric fever, gastroenteritis, grouping done on the basis of O and H antigens, known as **Kauffmann-White scheme.**

All salmonellae are motile except *S. gallinarum pullorum.*

All salmonellae are citrate positive except typhi and paratyphi A.

All salmonellae are citrate positive except paratyphi A.

Enteric fever diagnosed best by blood culture (especially first week), Widal (late second week, especially paired serum samples and fourfold rise in titer), stool culture (especially third week) or urine (fourth week or carriers). Typhi has only human-to-human transmission.

***Proteus***: show **swarming**, are **PPA** test positive.

***Shigella***: causes bacillary dysentery, all members of Family Enterobacteriaceae are catalase test positive except *Shigella dysenteriae* type 1.

**Oxidase positive** gram-negative bacilli:

***Vibrio:*** rice water stool, darting motility, oil drop appearance on Bile salt agar. Commonest vibrio: *V. cholerae* O1 Ogawa el Tor. *V. cholerae* O139 is known as **Bengal** strain.

## Pseudomonads

*Pseudomonas aeruginosa*: associated with bluish green pus and burn wound infections.

*Burkholderia mallei:* glanders, non-motile

*Burkolderia pseudomallei*: meliodosis, safety pin appearance, mimics plague, known as the Great Mimic.

*Burkholderia cepacia*: causes pulmonary infections in cystic fibrosis patients.

*Stenotrophomonas maltophila*: oxidase negative.

***Brucella***: causes brucellosis, zoonotic infection, prozone phenomenon seen (excessive production of antibodies).

***Bordetella***: causes pertussis or whooping cough, prevented by Killed whole cell vaccine which also acts as an adjuvant.

***Hemophilus***: *H. influenzae* type b most important in meningitis. Shows satellitism, Polysaccharide Hib vaccine used.

***Helicobacter:*** *H. pylori* associated with gastritis, ulcers, gastric carcinoma, atherosclerosis. Urea breath test done.

## Organisms that do not take up Gram Stain

**Mycobacteria:**

*M. tuberculosis* shows rough tough and buff colonies on LJ medium. ZN staining shows acid-fast bacilli.

*M. tuberculosis* is strongly acid-fast (can resist upto 20% $H_2SO_4$).

*M. leprae* is non-cultivable, grown in foot pad of mice or nine banded armadillo.

MOTT or NTM increasingly associated with immunocompromised state.

***Mycoplasma***: lack cell wall, show fried egg colonies.

***Chlamydia***: noncultivable, grown on McCoy cell line, cause trachoma, LGV, psittacosis, nongonococcal urethritis.

**Spirochetes:**

***Treponema pallidum***: causes syphilis. Primary stage shows chancre, which is painless. Organisms can be demonstrated from the chancre by darkfield microscopy. Diagnosis by serological tests. Standard tests for syphilis based on cardiolipin antigen, VDRL is screening test, 100% sensitive in secondary syphilis, prognostic significance as VDRL becomes negative after treatment. Specific tests based on treponemal antigen: Best specificity shown by *Treponema pallidum* immobilization (TPI) test, best sensitivity shown by FTA-Abs test. Routinely done test is TPHA.

***Borrelia***:

*B. recurrentis*: relapsing fever

*B. burgdorferi*: Lyme disease

*B. vincenti*: Vincent's angina

***Leptospira***: transmitted by rat urine.

**Rickettsiae**:

*R. prowazekii* – Epidemic typhus.

*R. typhi* - Endemic typhus.

*R. akari* – Rickettsial pox.

*R. rickettsii*–Rocky mountain spotted fever.

*R. tsutsugamushi* – Scrub typhus.

*Bartonella* (previously *Rochalemea*) *quintana* – Trench fever.

*Bartonella bacilliformis*–Bacillary angiomatosis.

*Bartonella henselae*–Cat scratch disease.

*Coxiella burnetii*–Q fever.

CHAPTER EIGHT

# Practice Questions

1. **One of the most remarkable aspects of the human immune system is its diversity, that is, the ability to recognize a wide range of antigens and to mount a specific antibody response. This is called "clonal selection." At the cellular level, which of the following are primarily responsible for such specificity?**
   a. Cytotoxic T cells
   b. Hypervariable regions in domains of B cells
   c. The major histocompatibility complex
   d. Specific T cell receptors
   e. Memory cells

2. **A young girl has repeated infections with *Candida albicans* and respiratory viruses since the time she was 3 months old. As part of the clinical evaluation of her immune status, her responses to routine immunization procedures should be tested. In this evaluation, the used of which of the following vaccines is contraindicated?**
   a. Diphtheria toxoid
   b. Bordetella pertussis vaccine
   c. Tetanus toxoid
   d. BCG
   e. Inactivated polio

3. **A latent, measles-like viral infection and, presumably a defect in cellular immunity is associated with which of the following diseases?**

a. Progressive multifocal leukoencephalopathy (PML)
b. Multiple sclerosis
c. Creutzfeldt-Jakob disease
d. Subacute sclerosing panencephalitis
e. Epstein-Barr virus infection

4. **In humans, two closely linked genetic loci, each made up of two alleles, compose the histocompatibility locus A (HL-A). Paired first and second locus antigens are called haplotypes. The HL-A haplotypes (separated by a semicolon) of a child's parents are given below. Father 3, 25; 7, 12. Mother 1, 3; 8, 9. Assuming that no cross-over events have occurred, the child's histotype could be which of the following?**
   a. 1, 3; 7, 8
   b. 7, 12; 1, 3
   c. 3, 3; 7, 9
   d. 1, 25; 7, 12
   e. 3, 25; 7, 12

5. **Immunity may be natural or acquired. Which of the following best describes acquired immunity?**
   a. Increase in C-reactive protein (CRP)
   b. Presence of natural killer (NK) cells
   c. Complement cascade
   d. Maternal transfer of antibody
   e. Inflammatory response

6. **Antigens can best be processed for presentation by:**
   a. Macrophages
   b. Kupffer cells
   c. B cells
   d. Young erythrocytes
   e. Suppressor T cells

7. **The best method for assessing the total number of B lymphocytes is:**
   a. QUANTITATIVE immunoglobulin levels
   b. Fc receptor assay

c. E rosette assay
d. Surface immunoglobulin (sIg) assay
e. Phytohemagglutinin A (PHA) mitogenicity

8. **Functional assessment of T lymphocyte includes:**
   a. E rosette assay
   b. Surface immunoglobulin (sIg) evaluation
   c. Transformation of lymphocytes by phytohemagglutinin A (PHA)
   d. Serum immunoglobulin determination
   e. Enumeration of theta-bearing cells

9. **After eating a dinner of leftovers that included rewarmed vegetable fried rice, a 17-year-old boy develops diarrhea and stomach pain. Which of the following is the most likely pathogen?**
   a. *Bacillus cereus*
   b. *Campylobater jejuni*
   c. *Clostridium botulinum*
   d. *Clostridium difficile*
   e. *Escherichia coli*

10. **A 3-year-old boy presents with a 1-day history of loose stools, fever, abdominal cramping, headache, and myalgia. He has no blood in the stool. A careful history reveals that he has several pet turtless. Which of the following is the most likely pathogen?**
    a. *Chlamydia psittaci*
    b. *Entamoeba histolytica*
    c. *Salmonella spp.*
    d. *Staphylococcus aureus*
    e. *Yersinia enterocolitica*

11. **A 22-year-old man gives blood samples for testing. Serum analysis yields elevated ALT, HBsAg, IgM Anti-HBc, HBeAg, and bilirubin. What is the hepatitis B status of this person?**
    a. Acute hepatitis
    b. Chronic persistent carrier
    c. Recovered from acute self-limited HBV
    d. Vaccinated against HBV

12. **Last year's influenza A vaccine is unlikely to be effective today because influenza A:**
    a. Has a heavy polysaccharide coat
    b. Immunosuppresses the patient
    c. Kills lymphocytes
    d. Resists inactivation by complement
    e. Undergoes genetic reassortment

13. **An 18-year-old, previously healthy woman presents to the student health service with fever, vomiting, and diarrhea. On physical examination, she is hypotensive and has an erythematous, red, sunburn like skin rash. She is currently menstruating and has been using super-absorbent tampons. Which of the following findings from a positive blood culture would confirm the suspected diagnosis?**
    a. Organisms are acid-fast
    b. Organisms are coagulase positive
    c. Organisms grow on EMB (eosin methylene blue) agar
    d. Organisms grow on Thayer-Martin media
    e. Organisms have positive Quellung reaction

14. **A 47-year-old man presents with a nonproductive cough and rales on his chest examination. A chest X-ray film suggests atypical pneumonia. The pneumonia resolves after treatment with azithromycin. A diagnosis of psittacosis is established by the presence of complement fixing antibodies against *Chlamydia psittaci* in the convalescent serum. Which of the following is the most likely occupation of this patient?**
    a. Cat breeder
    b. Florist
    c. Homeless shelter worker
    d. Poultry farmer
    e. Slaughterhouse worker

**15. Which of the following organisms is/are associated with manifestations of "immune complex" disease?**

a. *Plasmodium malariae*
b. *Streptococcus pyogenes*, group A
c. Hepatitis B virus
d. *Haemophilus influenaze*, type B

**16. "L-form" phenomenon is responsible for evading action of drugs mainly in:**

a. Mycobacterium tuberculosis
b. Pseudomonas
c. Proteus
d. Pasturella

**17. Exotoxins are produced by:**

a. Gram-negative bacilli
b. Gram-positive bacilli
c. Gram-negative cocci
d. Any of the above

**18. 'Fried egg' colony appearances of:**

a. *Mycobacterium leprae*
b. *Yersinia pestis*
c. *Mycoplasma*
d. *Proteus*

**19. Antisera are sterilized by:**

a. Autoclave
b. Hot air oven
c. Filtration
d. Steam under low pressure

**20. Which is not a test for syphilis?**

a. TPHA
b. Frei's test
c. Dark ground microscopy
d. RPR

**21. *Haemophilus ducreyi* is causastive agent of:**

a. Hard chancre
b. Soft chancre
c. Lymphogranuloma venereum
d. Granuloma inguinale

**22. Septicaemic spread of bacteria is the cause of the following diseases, *except*:**
a. Enteric fever
b. Diphtheria
c. Bacterial endocarditis
d. Miliary tuberculosis
e. Brucellosis

**23. False about typhoid fever is:**
a. Invariably comes originally from a human source
b. May be contracted from shellfish
c. Is caused by bacilli which multiply in the duodenum
d. Is easily diagnosed by blood culture on the third or fourth week
e. May cause lesions of Peyer's Patches

**24. Greenish discharge from a wound is most likely due to:**
a. *Staphylococcus*
b. *Esc. coli*
c. *Klebsiella*
d. *Pseudomonas*

**25. It has been hypothesized that there exists a strong association between hemolytic ureamic syndrome (HUS) and:**
a. *Salmonella*
b. Bacterophages of *Corynebacterium*
c. Verocytotoxin producing *Esch. coli* (VTEC)
d. *Clostridium diffcile*

**26. Staphylococcal food poisoning is caused by:**
a. Bacterial spores
b. Preformed exotoxin
c. Multiplication of bacteria
d. Preformed endotoxin

**27. Culture media useful for *Chlamydia* is:**
a. Sabouraud's medium
b. McLeod's medium
c. McCoy cell culture
d. Campy BAP medium

**28. An HIV-positive patient asks you if you can tell him the chances of him progressing to symptomatic AIDS. Which one of the following tests would be most useful?**

a. CD4 lymphocyte count
b. HIV antibody test
c. HIV RT PCR
d. Neopterin
e. HIV p24 antigen

**29. Griffith experiment proved:**

a. *Conjugation*
b. *Transformation*
c. Transduction
d. Transposon

**30. In which of the following is the genome doubled-stranded nucleic acid?**

a. Orthomyxoviruses
b. Poxviruses
c. Paroviruses
d. Reoviruses

**31. Hepatitis A virus is an enterovirus of type:**

a. Enterovirus 68
b. Enterovirus 69
c. Enterovirus 70
d. Enterovirus 71
e. Enterovirus 72

**32. Which of the following does not cause conjunctivitis?**

a. Adenovirus
b. Enterovirus
c. Coxsackie virus
d. Herpes virus

**33. The commonest cause of acute bronchiolitis is:**

a. Adenovirus
b. Respiratory syncytial virus
c. Mycoplasma
d. *H. influenzae*

34. **Which of the following is a DNA virus?**
   a. Polio type I
   b. Polio type II
   c. Rota virus
   d. Adenovirus

35. **Hepatitis E virus is best diagnosed by:**
   a. IgM antibodies in serum
   b. Immune electron microscopy on stool
   c. Culture from stool
   d. Isolation from bile

36. **Demateceous fungi are:**
   a. Produced in granules
   b. Intracellular parasites
   c. Brown
   d. Coenocytic

37. **Which viral infection always causes clinical disease in human beings?**
   a. Rubella
   b. Poliomyelitis
   c. Chickenpox
   d. Rabies

38. **Most fungi live as:**
   a. Animal parasites
   b. Parasites of trees and other vegetations
   c. Saprophytes
   d. Normal flora in man

39. **Phagocytosis of *C. neoformans* is inhibited by:**
   a. Cryptococcal capsular material
   b. The size of the yeast cells
   c. The cell walls
   d. Toxins produced by the organisms

40. **Hair perforation test is positive in infection with:**
   a. Trichophyton
   b. Microsporum
   c. Epidermophyton
   d. All of the above

41. **All of the following are dimorphic fungi *except*:**
    a. *Sporotrichum schenckii*
    b. *Cryptococcus neoformans*
    c. *Coccidiodes immitis*
    d. *Histoplasma capsulatum*

42. **The following are superficial fungal diseases *except*:**
    a. Pityriasis versicolor
    b. Dermatophytosis
    c. Piedra
    d. Mucomycosis

43. **Members of the genus *Candida* reproduce by:**
    a. Arthrospore formation
    b. Blastospore formation
    c. Sexual spores
    d. Ascospore formation

44. **Sclerotic bodies 3 – 15 m in size, multiseptate, chestnut brown color are seen in:**
    a. Rhinosporidiosis
    b. Chromoblastomycosis
    c. Phaeohyphomycosis
    d. Histoplasmosis

45. ***Cysticercus cellulosae* is seen in infection with:**
    a. *T. solium*
    b. *T. saginata*
    c. *Echinococcus*
    d. None of the above

46. **Definitive host for Guinea worm is:**
    a. Cyclops
    b. Man
    c. Cyclops and man
    d. Snail

47. **NIH swab is used for collection of specimen in:**
    a. Ankylostomiasis
    b. Ascariasis
    c. Taeniasis
    d. Enterobiasis

**48. For cutaneous larva migrans, humans are:**
a. Natural hosts
b. Aberrant hosts
c. Accidental hosts
d. None of the above

**49. Cat is an agent for transmission of the following disease to man:**
a. Isopora hominis
b. Fasciola hepatica
c. Toxoplasma gondii
d. Chilomastic mensili

**50. Which of the following parasite has the appearance of a tennis racket with a concave ventral surface?**
a. *Balantidium coli*
b. *Giardia intestinalis*
c. *Trichomonas*
d. *Entamoeba histolytica*

**51. The worms which may be found in muscles are:**
a. Trichinella
b. Taenia saginata
c. Taenia sodium
d. All of above

**52. The following tests help in laboratory diagnosis of kala azar *except*:**
a. Bone marrow examination
b. Immobilisation test
c. Blood smear examination
d. Aldehyde test

**53. Largest intestinal protozoa is:**
a. *Entamoeba coli*
b. *Balantidium coli*
c. *Giardia lamblia*
d. *Toxoplasma gondii*

**54. The drug of choice for dermal, oral and vaginal candidiasis is:**
a. Griseofulvin
b. Amphotericin B

c. Gentian violet
d. Nystain

**55. Killed bacterial vaccine is:**
a. BCG
b. Yellow fever
c. Pertussis
d. Colchicins

**56. Live attenuated vaccine of influenza is given:**
a. Orally
b. Intramuscularly
c. Subcutaneously
d. Intranasally

**57. Bacille Calmette Guerin (BCG) contains the avirulent strains of:**
a. Human tubercle bacilli
b. Avian tubercle bacilli
c. Bovine tubercle bacilli
d. Atypical mycobacteria

**58. Which of the following vaccine is also for stimulating immune system?**
a. BCG
b. DPT
c. Measles
d. Polio

**59. Anti-HBs antibodies indicates:**
a. Good prognosis
b. Hepatocellular Ca
c. Resistance to Hepatitis B
d. Acute infection

**60. Rabies virus can multiply in:**
a. The central nervous system only
b. The peripheral nerves
c. Muscle tissue
d. Connective tissues
e. All the above

**61. Which of the following is/are known to exist in only one major antigenic type *except*?**
a. Measles
b. Rubella

c. Mumps
d. Adenovirus

62. **Dengue spread by:**
a. Anopheles
b. Culex
c. Mansoides
d. Aedes

63. **The live vaccines are available against the following viruses *except*:**
a. Influenza
b. Measles
c. Polio
d. Rabies

64. **When a laboratory animal is inoculated with one virus, the host cells may be protected against subsequent challenge with a second virus, this is known as:**
a. Haemagglutination
b. Haemadsorption
c. Moderate virus
d. Interference

65. **False about continuous cell lines:**
a. Capable of continuous serial multiplication
b. Used for virus isolation
c. Derived from cancer cells
d. Used for manufacture of viral vaccines

66. **Henderson-Peterson bodies are seen infection due to:**
a. Smallpox
b. Fowlpox
c. Molluscum contagiosum
d. Rabies

67. **Brick-shaped virus is:**
a. Rhabdovirus
b. Reovirus
c. Orthomyxovirus
d. Vaccinia virus

68. **Myocarditis is caused by:**
a. Influenza virus

b. Measles virus
c. Coxsackie B
d. Epstein Barr virus

**69. Which of the following virus produces both intranuclear and intracytoplasmic antibodies?**
a. Rabies
b. Herpes
c. Measles
d. Polio virus

**70. All of the following are properties of virus *except*:**
a. Highly infective
b. Host specificity
c. Tissue specificity or cytotropism
d. Lowly antigenic

**71. All of the following viruses are segmented *except*:**
a. Orthomyxovirus
b. Paramyxovirus
c. Bunyavirus
d. Arenavirus

**72. The staining useful for antemortem diagnosis of rabies is:**
a. Seller
b. Macchiavillo
c. Giemsa
d. Fluorescent

**73. Which of the following virus can be seen by light microscopy?**
a. Vaccinia
b. Hepatitis
c. Herpes
d. Reovirus

**74. Aplastic crisis in sickle cell anemia is associated with:**
a. Parvovirus B-19
b. SV-40
c. Arenavirus
d. Rubella virus

75. **Monoclonal antibodies are:**
   a. More sensitive than conventional antisera
   b. Produced by a single clone of T lymphocytes
   c. Secreted by myeloma-thymic lymphocyte hybridoma
   d. Formed at a single class of immunoglobulins
   e. All of the above

76. **The number of bacterial cell is increased in:**
   a. Lag phase
   b. Exponential phase
   c. Acceleration phase
   d. Stationary phase

77. **Anamnestic reaction is defined as:**
   a. Production of heterologous but related antibody in response to antigenic stimulation
   b. Selective proliferation of plasma cells produce antibodies
   c. A kind of primary immune response
   d. None of the above

78. **Agglutination reaction is:**
   a. Wasserman
   b. VDRL
   c. Kahn
   d. Widal

79. **Incomplete antibody gives:**
   a. Casoni's test
   b. Coombs' test
   c. Wasseman's test
   d. Frie's test

80. **Type I immediate hypersensitivity reaction is seen in:**
   a. Serum sickness
   b. Casoni's test
   c. Arthus reaction
   d. Immune complex disease

81. **True about sterilization is:**
   a. Spores are destroyed by drying
   b. Soiled dressing are sterilized by hot air oven
   c. Surgical instruments are sterilized by boiling
   d. Vaccines sterilized by Seitz filters

**82. One of the characteristics of arboviruses is that they:**

a. Are transmitted by arthropod vectors
b. Are usually resistant to ether
c. Usually cause symptomatic infection in humans
d. Are closely related to parvoviruses

**83. Echoviruses are cytopathogenic human viruses that mainly infect the:**

a. Respiratory system
b. Central nervous system
c. Blood and lymphatic systems
d. Intestinal tract
e. Bladder and urinary tract

**84. All of the following viruses may be human tumor viruses *except*:**

a. Epstein-Barr virus (EBV)
b. Human T cell leukemia virus (HTLV)
c. Papilloma virus
d. Varicella-zoster virus (VZV)
e. Herpes simplex virus, Type II (HSV)

**85. Interferon, a protein that inhibits viral replication, is produced by cells in tissue culture when the cells are stimulated with all the following *except:***

a. Endotoxin
b. Synthetic double-stranded polynucleotides
c. Viruses
d. Chlamydiae
e. Rickettsiae

**86. All of the following viral genomes are replicated in the cytoplasm *except*:**

a. Reoviruses
b. Picornaviruses
c. Poxviruses
d. Paramyxoviruses
e. Herpes viruses

**87. A 19-year-old college student developed a rash. She worked part time in a pediatric AIDS clinic. Her blood was drawn and tested**

**for specific antibody to the chickenpox virus (varicella-zoster). Which of the following antibody classes would you expect if she were immune to chickenpox?**

a. IgA
b. IgD
c. IgE
d. IgG
e. IgM

88. ***Candida albicans*** **is recognized in microscopic examination of infected tissues by the presence of:**

a. Spherules containing endospores
b. Metachromatic granules
c. Yeasts and pseudohyphae
d. Asci containing two-eight ascospores
e. Abundance of septate rhizoids

89. **The mechanism of mucosal invasion by *Candida albicans* is at least partially understood. Which one of the following modifications in the structure or function of this yeast would be most likely to affect its invasive ability?**

a. Loss of ability to produce ethanol from glucose
b. Loss of ability to produce germ tubes or hyphae
c. Reduced ability to grow at 37°C
d. Loss of ability to produce a polysaccharide capsule
e. Replaced of mannan in the cell wall with glucan

90. **Which of the following best describes an infection with *Coccidioides immitis*?**

a. A negative complement fixing (CF) antibody test
b. Inhaled arthrospores form thick walled spherules filled with endospores
c. "Fungus ball" formation
d. Thrush
e. Clavate macroconidia

91. **A gardener pricked his toe while cutting rose bushes. Four days later a pustule that changed to an ulcer developed on his toe. Then 3 modules formed along the local lymphatic drainage. The most likely agent is:**
   a. *Trichophyton rubrum*
   b. *Aspergillus fumigatus*
   c. *Candida albicans*
   d. *Sporothroix schenkii*
   e. *Cryptococcus neoformans*

92. **A 19-year-old girl has smooth, annular, scaly, erythematous, vesicular lesions on her leg. Assuming that you suspect corporis, what would be the most suitable laboratory diagnostic approach?**
   a. Silver staining of tissue scrappinig
   b. Acid-fast staining on the vesicular fluid
   c. Culture of the vesicular fluid on agar
   d. Digestion of tissue biopsies with 10-20% KOH
   e. Serology for *Blastomyces dermatitidis*

93. **Which of the following statements about host defenses against fungal infections is/are not correct?**
   a. Antibody is not protective
   b. Leukocytes can kill fungi
   c. Mild illness can confer protection against future infections
   d. Interferon released from lymphocytes slows fungal metabolism

94. **Asexual spores of fungi are following *except*:**
   a. Arthrospores
   b. Chlamydospores
   c. Blastospores
   d. Ascospores

95. ***Cryptococcus neoformans* has been found growing most often in:**
   a. Water
   b. Soil containing pigeon feces
   c. Chicken feces
   d. Desert soils

**96. The medium of choice for culturing the yeast from of dimorphic fungi is:**
a. Brain-heart infusion
b. Sabouraud's
c. Sabouraud's plus antibodies
d. Any medium incubated at 35-37°C

**97. Which is not true of *Cryptococcus neoformans*?**
a. Grows at 37°C
b. Grows on Sabouraud's agar
c. Polysaccharide capsule
d. Urease negative

**98. Vascular involvement and thrombosis is seen in:**
a. *Mucormycosis*
b. *Coccidioidomycosis*
c. *Aspergillosis*
d. None

**99. Which of the following shows tumbling motility?**
a. *Vibrio cholerae*
b. *Salmonella*
c. *Shigella*
d. *Listeria*
e. *Spirochetes*

**100. Which of the following is oxidase test negative?**
a. *Helicobacter*
b. *Brucella*
c. *E. coli*
d. *Vibrio*
e. *Pseudomonas*

## ANSWERS AND EXPLANATIONS

1. (b) Humoral response is governed by B cells and diversity is due to hypervariable regions
2. (d) Repeated *Candida* infection depicts immunocompromised state and live attenuated vaccines are contraindicated in such individuals.
3. (d) SSPE is a post-measles complication associated with defective cellular immunity.
4. (b) As crossing over hasn't occurred, the pairs will stay together, i.e. father can give either 3,25 or 7,12 to the child and no other combination. Similarly mother can transfer 1,3 or 8,9. No other choice fulfills this condition.
5. (d) This is a type of passive acquired immunity since the child is not producing antibodies on its own but getting readymade antibodies from mother.
6. (a) Although various types of cells can act as antigen presenting cells (APCs), amongst the choices macrophages are the best.
7. (d) Quantitation can be done by surface markers assay.
8. (c) This is a test for qualitative assessment for T cells.
9. (a) Stale Chinese food can result in *B. cereus* infection.
10. (c) *Salmonella* species inhabit and infect varied host animals including reptiles, birds, mammals and aquatic animals while other choices have limited host range.
11. (b) Presence of IgM anti-HBc depicts acute infection. HBsAg depicts infection, HbeAg depicts infectivity.
12. (e) Segmented orthomyxovirus has a predilection to get reassorted changing the antigenic character.
13. (b) Clinical features and use of tampon points towards toxic shock syndrome (TSS) caused mainly by *Staphylococcus aureus*, which are coagulase positive.

14. (d) Psittacosis is associated with birds.
15. (b) Post-streptococcal glomerulonephritis and rheumatic fever are immune complex mediated complications of Group A streptococci.
16. (a) Antitubercular drugs do not have much action on L-forms (cell wall deficient) so that mycobacteria can survive in the host.
17. (d) Endotoxins are a part of gram-negative cell wall whereas any type of bacteria can produce exotoxin.
18. (c) Typical appearance with dark center and light surroundings like fried egg, seen under light microscope after staining.
19. (c) Heat sensitive therefore neither dry nor moist heat can be used.
20. (b)
21. (a)
22. (b) Diphtheria is a result of toxemia, i.e. spread of toxin and bacteria remain localized in the throat.
23. (b) *S. typhi* has no non-human host.
24. (d) *Pseudomonas aeruginosa* produces various pigments most importantly pathognomic greenish pigment. Non-pigmented pseudomonas strains also occur.
25. (c) HUS is associated with various organisms- *Shigella*, VTEC/EHEC, *Campylobacter*.
26. (b) Bacteria usually not found in remaining food particles implicated in food poisoning as get killed during cooking, but toxin remains and can be detected.
27. (c) *Chlamydia* cannot be grown *in vitro*, but can be grown in McCoy cell lines.
28. (c) Quantitation of the viral load is the best prognostic indicator
29. (b) Naked DNA is the carrier of genetic information in transformation, proven by Griffith experiment
30. (d) Reoviridae is the only RNA virus group of human importance that are double-stranded.

Also Parvoviridae is the only DNA virus group of human importance that are single-stranded.

31. (e) Recently has been reclassified separately as Hepatovirus under Picornaviridae.
32. (d) Causes keratitis
33. (b) Occurs mainly in children.
34. (d)
35. (b) Can be visualized in stool by electron microscopy.
36. (c) Also known as back moulds, usually laboratory contaminants but can cause opportunistic infections especially keratitis. Examples are *Curvalaria, Alternaria*, etc. Coenocytic means aseptate, e.g. *Mucor, Rhizopus*.
37. (d) Rabies carrier state in humans is not known. Infection always leads to disease.
38. (c) Usually fungi are inhabitants of soil and invade humans as opportunists. Dermatophytes are the only true obligate fungal pathogens.
39. (a) Most of the meningitis causing organisms including fungus like Cryptococcus and bacteria like pneumococci, meningococci and Hemophilus are capsulated.
40. (a) Hair perforation test is used for distinguishing Trichophyton rubrum from *T. mentagrophytes*. *T. rubrum* is positive for this test. Hair baiting is a test used to select out dermatophytes from soil.
41. (b) Present as yeast only.
42. (d) Mucormycosis is a systemic infection with predilection for endothelial cells of capillaries and results in thromboembolic episodes and may lead to DIC.
43. (b) Reproduction of yeast cell by blast formation or pinching off of new cell is called blastospore formation. Arthrospore seen in, e.g. Trichosporon, Ascospore is a sexual spore seen in, e.g. *Aspergillus*.
44. (b) Also known as muriform cells. Distinguishing feature from Phaeohyphomycosis.

45. (a)
46. (b) Man is a definite host for almost all parasites except *Echinococcus* and *Plasmodium*.
47. (d) Used to collect eggs deposited by the female worm in the perianal area of host.
48. (b)
49. (c)
50. (b) Trophozoite of Giardia has this typical shape.
51. (d) Some form either adult or larvae of all these may be found in muscles.
52. (b) Most specific test done for syphilis.
53. (b) Also the only ciliate to cause human infection.
54. (d) Used for topical application.
55. (c) P component in DPT is killed pertussis, which also functions as an adjuvant.
56. (d) Provides local immunity also as this is the natural route of entry of influenza virus.
57. (c)
58. (a) Also functions as immunomodulator.
59. (c) Presence of HBsAg depicts resistance to infection, could be following natural infection and recovery or following vaccination.
60. (e) Although the primary tissue of multiplication is nervous tissue, multiplication can also occur to a large extent in muscle and connective tissues.
61. (d) Adenovirus has at least 42 antigenic types and they can cause varied disease presentations.
62. (d) Vector is Aedes species.
63. (d) This is a universally fatal infection and reverting back to wild form by attenuated strain is too big a risk to allow live vaccines to be tried.
64. (d) This is especially seen with Rubella with which adenovirus cause interference.
65. (d) Possibility that transfer of tumor antigens may lead to malignant changes.
66. (c)

67. (d) Poxviruses are brick-shaped and rabies virus is bullet-shaped.
68. (c)
69. (c) Generally viruses produce either intranuclear or in cytoplasmic inclusions depending on their site of replication. Measles is an exception.
70. (d) Viruses result in tremendous immune response although it may or may not be protective.
71. (b) Apart from these Reovirus group is also segmented.
72. (d)
73. (a) Poxviruses are the largest viruses.
74. (a) Also causes fifth disease characterized by erythema in slapped cheek appearance
75. (e) New method of producing monoclonal antibodies is called phage display technique.
76. (b) This phase is also called log phase with maximum or logarithmic growth.
77. (a) Can lead to false positivity in serological tests, e.g. positive Widal test after viral infection due to previous infection of typhoid bacteria.
78. (d) Widal is tube flocculation, Wasserman is complement fixation, VDRL is slide flocculation and Kahn is tube flocculation.
79. (b) Coombs' test done for Rh incompatibility in mother and fetus.
80. (b) Anaphylactic reaction is type I hypersensitivity.
81. (d) Heat sensitive fluids may be sterilized by filtration.
82. (a) **Ar**- arthropod **bo**- borne.
83. (b) **E**- enteric **C**- cytopathogenic **H**- human **O**-orphan viruses commonly cause aseptic meningitis.
84. (d) Causes chickenpox or herpes zoster.
85. (a) Interferon production induced by viruses or other intracellular organisms and not endotoxin.
86. (e) Poxviruses as an exception are the only DNA viruses to replicate in the cytoplasm.

87. (d) IgM depicts recent infection whereas IgG indicates post-exposure and immunity.
88. (c) Pseudohyphae indicate invasion by *Candida.*
89. (b)
90. (b) Spherules and arthroconidia are characteristic features.
91. (d) Usually subcutaneous infection following thorn prick or vegetative matter injury.
92. (d) Done for dermatophytic infections to clear off keratin.
93. (c) There is no protective immunity to natural fungal infections.
94. (d) Sexual spores are mainly ascospores, basidiospores and zygospores.
95. (b) Can survive in high temperatures of birds.
96. (a) Conditions including temperature similar to *in vivo* conditions
97. (d) Urease positive—used as a test for identification.
98. (a) Systemic infection by Mucor, now also known as zygomycosis.
99. (d) Listeria has amphitrichous flagellae
100. (c) *E. coli* belongs to Enterobacteriaceae family which is oxidase negative